DISCARDED BY
MEMPHIS PUBLIC LIBRARY

VITAL information

What you need to know ABOUT

HMOs and The Patient's Bill of Rights

BY MOLLY SHAPIRO, R.N., M.S., M.B.A., Ed.D.

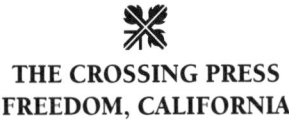

THE CROSSING PRESS
FREEDOM, CALIFORNIA

*This book is dedicated to
Bernard and Isabell Rubel*

Copyright © 1999 by Molly Shapiro
Cover design by Victoria May
Interior design by Magnolia Studio
Printed in the U.S.A.

All rights reserved.

The information contained in this book is not intended as a substitute for consulting with your physician or other health care provider. Any attempt to diagnose and treat an illness should be done under the direction of a health care professional. The publisher does not advocate the use of any particular health care protocol, but believes that the information in this book should be available to the public. The publisher and author are not responsible for any adverse effects or consequences resulting from the use of any of the suggestions, preparations, or procedures discussed in this book.

No part of this publication may be reproduced or transmitted in any form or by any means, electric or mechanical, including photocopy, recording, or any information storage and retrieval system now known or to be invented, without permission in writing from the publisher, except by a reviewer who wishes to quote brief passages in connection with a review written for inclusion in a magazine, newspaper, or broadcast. Contact The Crossing Press, Inc., P.O Box 1048, Freedom, CA 95019.

For information on bulk purchases or group discounts for this and other Crossing Press titles, please contact our Special Sales Manager at 800-777-1048.

Visit our Web site on the Internet: **www.crossingpress.com**

Library of Congress Cataloging-in-Publication Data

Shapiro, Molly, RN.
    HMOs and the patient's bill of rights / by Molly Shapiro.
        p. cm. -- (Vital information)
    Includes bibliographical references and index.
    ISBN 1-58091-024-6 (pbk.)
    1. Health maintenance organizations--United States. 2. Patients-
-Legal status, laws, etc.--United States. 3. Right to health care-
-United States. I. Title. II. Series.
RA413.5.U5S53   1999
362.1'04258--dc21   99-36402
                                                                                                CIP

Contents

INTRODUCTION: WHY A BILL OF RIGHTS? 7

CHAPTER 1: **WHAT PROMPTED THE HMO CONCEPT?** 9
Consumerism
History
Diagnostic Related Groupings or DRGs
Downsizing in Health Care
A Crowded Playing Field

CHAPTER 2: **WHAT IS YOUR RIGHT TO HEALTH CARE AS A MANAGED CARE PATIENT?**
Is Health Care a Right or an Individual Responsibility? .16
Americans Who Have a Right to Health Care
Americans Who Have a Responsibility for Health Care
Universal Access
A Federal Bill of Rights for HMO Patients
A State Bill of Rights for HMO Patients
Which Move Affects Who?

CHAPTER 3: **WHO ARE THE PLAYERS?** 22
Rational Behavior
When One Change Affects Many
Integrated Health Care Networks
The Demand for Health Care

CHAPTER 4: **ON WHOSE SIDE ARE PROVIDER GROUPS? How Is Your Doctor Thinking?** 27
Catch-Up Economics
Power Shifts from Physicians to HMOs
Provider-Sponsored HMOs
Physician-Sponsored Hospitals
Conceptual Flaws
Accountability
Added Complexities
Cooperative Care
Advantages of Cooperative Care
Disadvantages

CHAPTER 5: ON WHOSE SIDE IS THE HOSPITAL SYSTEM?
How Are Treatment Centers Thinking? 38
Hospital Networks
Advantages of Hospital Networks
Conceptual Flaws
A Different Mission: Research and Education
Scarce Health Care Resources
Scarce Human Resources
Balancing Yin and Yang

CHAPTER 6: ON WHOSE SIDE IS YOUR STATE?
On Whose Side Is Your Employer? 44
State Innovations
How Much Is Too Much?
Legislators' Interests
Conceptual Flaws
One State's Solution
Conceptual Flaws
For You to Get Rights, You Will Pay More than Your Share
Conclusion

CHAPTER 7: ON WHOSE SIDE IS YOUR HMO OR OTHER MANAGED CARE ORGANIZATION? .53
Economies of Scale
Managed Competition
Conceptual Flaws
The Challenge
Monitors

CHAPTER 8: ON WHOSE SIDE IS YOUR CASE MANAGER? And How Is Care Managed? 63
History
Seamless Support
Protocols
Outcomes Mandated by the NCQA
How to Take More Responsibility in Your Care
Holding Treatment Centers Accountable
Disadvantages of Case Managers
Advantages of Case Managers
Conceptual Flaws
Conclusion

CHAPTER 9:   ON WHOSE SIDE IS
             THE FEDERAL GOVERNMENT?
             How Is Rationing Used? 72
             Federal Goals
             Asymmetric Information
             Supply and Demand
             Rationing
             Rationing that Increases Supply
             Advantages of Nurses as Primary Care Providers
             Disadvantages of Nurses as Primary Care Providers
             Increasing Competition in Health Care
             Myths and Rebuttals to Diluting Care
             What Happens If HMOs Are Forced to Take on High-
                Risk Patients?

CHAPTER 10: WHERE DO YOU DRAW THE LINE?
             What About Standards or Quality Care? 84
             Drawing Boundaries in Efficiency and Equity
             Drawing Boundaries in Outcome Measures
             Challenges in Collecting Outcomes
             Acknowledging Adverse Outcomes
             Long-Term Effects
             Other Long-Term Implications
             Drawing Legal Boundaries
             Drawing Ethical Boundaries
             Drawing Boundaries in Protocols
             Conclusion

CHAPTER 11: HOW IS MANAGED CARE CREATING
             PROGRESS? Why Is Health Care For-Profit? ..94
             Implications
             A Lesson Learned from Canada
             Making Organ Donation Self-Sufficient
             Making Organ Donation Profitable
             Advantages
             Disadvantages
             Conclusion

CHAPTER 12: WHAT ARE ALTERNATIVE SOLUTIONS? 101
             Removing Conflict of Interest for Providers
             Provider-Sponsored HMOs
             Patient Determined Rationing with Medical Savings
                Accounts (MSAs)
             Avoidance
             Geographically Specific Solutions
             The Moral Objective: Which Method Limits More Disease
                and Death?
             What Do Americans Want?
             Conclusion

CHAPTER 13: **WHAT HAPPENS AS THINGS CHANGE?** 125
Mergers and Acquisitions
Prevention
Consumer Awareness
Disease Management
Assisted Living
Too Much Change Too Fast
Alternative Therapies
Conclusion

CHAPTER 14: **HOW WILL MANAGED CARE HURT PROGRESS?** 131
Winners and Losers
Designer Drugs: Statins and Viagra
Who Gets Designer Drugs?
Costs of Designer Drugs in Health Care
Consumer Sovereignty
Conceptual Flaws in CEA
Economic Malpractice

CHAPTER 15: **SO WHAT HAPPENS NEXT?**
What Does the Future Hold? 142
Information Technology
Convenience in Health Care
Quality of Life Issues
Consumers Demand Accountability
Cost Constraints Spawn New Models
Predictions for the Future of Health Care

CHAPTER 16: **WHAT ARE YOUR RIGHTS?** 150
A New Health Care Bill of Rights
The Theory of Regulation
Who Should Ration Your Care?
Coming Full Circle: Consumerism

INDEX 156

Why a Bill of Rights?

Do you wonder how Health Maintenance Organizations (HMOs), providers, hospitals, and bureaucrats can behave so recklessly? It is because we, the people, are not involved in health care decisions. Health plans are chosen by employers, or the government if you belong to Medicare or Medicaid HMOs. The same is true of doctors, provider groups, and hospital networks. They are chosen for you. Therefore, you are not the customer. And that is why no one listens to you anymore. Now, the customers in health care are employers and the government. Employers buy your benefits as an employee, and governments buy benefits for the elderly or poverty patients. The less frills and the cheaper the plan, all the better for them. If they are paying for your health care, then providers and hospitals do not have to please you, the patient. You cannot force the market to improve by taking your business elsewhere. Competition has been adulterated by current methods of managed care.

How is this happening? Health care costs grow out of control. Medicare and Medicaid are going bankrupt. Purposely, the government has enabled cost-cutting HMOs to dominate health care. But what is wrong with this picture? Legally, HMOs do not have enforceable standards for quality. And they are growing into—by definition—monopolies.

The government has power only because the people give it to them. If power lies with the people, a critical mass is needed to remind the government of whom they represent. Each time you vote, you are choosing someone to make your health care decisions. Is this how you want things to remain? Do elected officials have private health insurance and, as a result, have less concerns with their constituents' personal health care coverage? Yet we, the people, have the power. Therefore, we had better learn who the decision-makers are, how they think, and why. Then we can responsibly vote for change.

Health care can be confusing. No one side of health care has the whole truth. Much of your opinion will depend on to whom you talk and trust. As the author of this book, I am a nurse provider with an MBA who belongs to an HMO. I try to maintain a broad view. But there are many perspectives on HMOs, some of which I am ignorant. But when I use health care, I must consider reasons for certain behaviors. Your behavior, too, must be based on complex motives. An open mind is necessary to learn about the complexities of contemporary health care. It is true that there are flaws in our current system that need attention. But there is no one method of health care that is absolutely right or wrong. Your opinion will depend on who you are and where you stand.

The purpose of this book is to present more angles on HMOs, for whichever side of the side rails you may be standing. And it is an attempt to let the buyer—and seller of health care—beware. My goal is to create awareness, and to stimulate controversy and change. I invite you to share and meet these goals.

CHAPTER 1

What Prompted the HMO Concept?

> *"Today's health care consumer is a sleeping giant—one who is awakening to his power. Fully awakened, he will be the master and health care providers will be the servants."*
> —Leland R. Kaiser, *Health Care's Sleeping Giant*

The mighty pen of Mr. Kaiser forecasts optimism. Unfortunately, many painful changes must occur before this prediction will materialize. We, as health care consumers, have a lot of work to do. But you may take comfort in knowing that efforts will be rewarded.

For our convenience, banks invented ATMs for access to cash 24 hours a day. Levi Strauss will make jeans based on your exact measurements. And Internet technology disseminates information with new speed and breadth. When industries pay attention to the needs of their consumers, they have customers for life.

CONSUMERISM

Congratulations, you were once a passive participant in the health care process. But you, the consumer, have become increasingly vocal in recent years. There are a number of ways you have been heard in the health care process.

- ▲ Challenging the health plans that deny treatment
- ▲ Fighting for legally mandated benefits
- ▲ Disenrolling and opting for plans that provide choice

- ▲ Demanding information about providers and quality of care and
- ▲ Demonstrating a readiness to shop and compare prices

Consumer momentum is shifting. If, when the dust settles, Congress makes a move, who will still be standing? Will it be health care entities with consumer-driven strategies? These are the "businesses" that sell products and services to consumers, and not bureaucratic-driven institutions.

OTHER CONSUMER AND LEGISLATIVE CONCERNS

- ▲ *Information Disclosure*
- ▲ *More Provider Choice*
- ▲ *Emergency Services*
- ▲ *Participation in Treatment Decisions*
- ▲ *Respect and Nondiscrimination*
- ▲ *Confidentiality of Health Information*
- ▲ *Complaints and Appeals Process*
- ▲ *Consumer Responsibilities*
- ▲ *ERISA*
- ▲ *Direct Access to Specialists*
- ▲ *Open Drug Formulary*
- ▲ *Access to Clinical Trials*
- ▲ *Gag Clause Ban*
- ▲ *Mastectomy Length of Stay Mandate*
- ▲ *Longer Maternity Length of Stay*

HISTORY

Once upon a time, in bureaucratic-driven health care, your doctors could order any test, procedure, or any pill for you. Your insurance would pick up the tab, no questions asked. Medicare paid the elderly's medical expenses, no questions asked. And Medicaid covered the medical expenses of the disabled and unsupported women and their children. This was the 1980s, when the majority of health care payment systems were called "fee-for-service." However, a financial free-for-all was occurring. Insurance companies began to get huge bills. They saw tests ordered that were not needed. Why? Because a few greedy doctors owned the laboratories and x-ray machines. They could make a lot of money by ordering more tests on every patient. These doctors could take advantage of this system with the power of their knowledge. They could argue that defensive medicine prevented lawsuits. And they were right. (Chapter 4 presents further perspectives of providers.)

In those days, hospitals had a similar advantage. They could house patients on an open tab for almost indefinitely. The longer patients stayed, the more hospitals could charge. Patients were discharged, not when they were well, but when they asked to go home. (The hospital perspective is addressed at length in Chapter 5.)

For those with more ideas than ethics, there was money to be made. Even patients could abuse the system. If health care was

WHAT IS DEFENSIVE MEDICINE?

Doctors are human and can make mistakes. And lawyers will take advantage of missed diagnoses. This leads providers to order many tests to rule out many diagnoses on patients with unknown illnesses. This may seem like common sense, but it is expensive—especially when someone else pays the bill and it occurs with more and more patients.

paid by others, then why not use the emergency room for a minor ache or rash? The system failed to discourage abuses. It was doing an average job, yet it required more and more money.

One day, the government woke up health care by placing spending limits on diagnoses.

DIAGNOSTIC RELATED GROUPINGS OR DRGS

A DRG is a fee that is "usual, customary, and reasonable" that represents the cost to treat an average patient suffering from an average diagnosis. All diagnoses were assigned price tags. With DRGs, the government stopped runaway billing for government patients. No matter how much was spent on Medicaid patients, doctors and hospitals were given billing caps.

For a procedure such as an appendectomy, facilities could bill for surgery plus the cost of two hospital days. For an illness such as asthma, a person needed two to three days in the hospital. This meant hospitals could bill for three days worth of care. No longer could patients stay in the hospital at the expense of taxpayers. At that time, the choice became: a limit with DRGs, or legislators would raise taxes. And taxpayers were not voting for officials who increased taxes.

The result of DRGs was drastic. These low reimbursement rates meant losses for hospitals who operated in Medicare communities. Since no money could be made from government patients, hospitals began to "cost-shift." This meant hospitals overinflated charges to hospitalized patients with health insurance. This extra money was generated to cover the losses of treating Medicare patients.

DOWNSIZING IN HEALTH CARE

Two things happened. First, many small hospitals closed. Those that treated rural elderly patients or that saw mostly Medicare patients could not afford to stay open. They did not have the opportunity, the shrewdness, or the conscience to cost-shift. In effect, DRGs closed hospitals who feared bad publicity, the very institutions with moral integrity and good will. (Chapter 5 addresses the hospital perspective at greater length.) Meanwhile, some provider groups tried to limit the number of Medicare patients in their practices. Later, this became discrimination.

Secondly, if the government could set limits, why couldn't insurance companies? Some companies began to review hospital bills carefully. And eventually, the insurance industry grasped onto the idea of dictating how medicine could practice.

Today, we feel the effects of limited health care coverage. Our generation gets to suffer through painful cutbacks. Perhaps the next generation will feel no pain, never having tasted the days of excess. However, it is important that this pain and passion be harnessed now. Having lived both extremes, we have more knowledge. This knowledge must be channeled to force a compromise—perhaps somewhere in the middle of fee-for-service and managed care.

Patients are doing their part in compromising. Here is how patients, doctors, and hospitals are compromising for their share of health care costs.

- ▲ Today, doctors cannot order unnecessary tests or unproven therapies without penalties.

- ▲ Hospitals must ration health care or absorb the costs. Hospitals cannot keep your mom through the weekend if you are inconvenienced by her illness.

- ▲ Patients go home sooner. Reports show you sleep better at home, when not awakened for blood pressure readings or sleeping pills. Modern patients are interested in learning about diseases and take more responsibility for recovery. Certainly, you can dispense your own medications as well as any nurse. But if you need a complicated dressing change or treatment, a nurse can come to your house. A home visit costs a fraction of one day in the hospital.

But how are HMOs doing their part at compromising? We know we are in the managed care era, where health care is streamlined. However, MCOs (Managed Care Organizations) manage patients, providers, hospitals, and other networks so tightly that everyone is tired of over compromising. Frustration and concern for quality has become a backlash from all involved.

A CROWDED PLAYING FIELD

Since managed care is somewhat complex, no one is quite sure how it should be regulated. Networks do not want to step on each other's toes. Meanwhile, the government is happy to delegate health care rationing headaches to big businesses. Then it can look the other way while appearing blameless. It does not have to raise more financial support through taxes. (The federal government's position is explored further in Chapter 9.)

Who is left? States could take up some of the slack. Actually, states are in a good position to take charge. States know best their differing populations with varying needs. Health care in rural Alaska cannot be managed with the same rules used in New York City. And some states are not yet deeply penetrated by managed care. (The states' position is developed in Chapter 6.)

INTEGRATED DELIVERY SYSTEMS

Exactly who is involved, and who is responsible to whom? The HMO acts as a funnel or a bottleneck. HMOs control health care because everyone must move through their web. (This perspective is further argued in Chapter 3.)

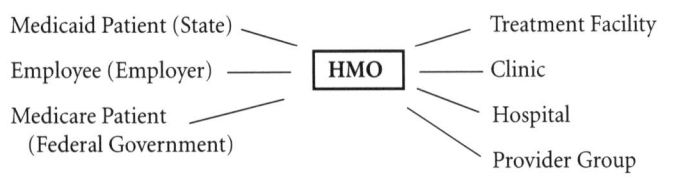

Employers have some power, too. A healthy labor force is maintained by looking out for their employees' best health interests. Employers can seek HMOs with excellent reputations and middle-of-the-road costs. This encourages higher standards. (Chapter 6 takes on this view.)

So the playing field is fairly crowded. You can see that establishing a patient's bill of rights is not mutually exclusive. The rippling effects of one small change will be felt by everyone identified above. A bill of rights with ten changes may create total chaos. Everyone has a different idea of what should change and who should pay for it. As you read about how each player thinks, you will begin to understand the magnitude of making changes. We need to consider carefully:

- ▲ what changes we need as opposed to what changes would be nice,
- ▲ how they will affect each player, and
- ▲ how the players could behave as a result.

References
Consumerism in Health Care: New Voices (1/98). KPMG.

CHAPTER 2

What Is Your Right to Health Care as a Managed Care Patient?

Is Health Care a Right or an Individual Responsibility?

First of all, what is a right? What is a responsibility? And what is our current system?

A right is, "something one has a just or lawful claim." (Merriam-Webster, 1998). In this context, health care must be provided for all. This is called universal coverage or even socialized medicine.

A responsibility is, "a liability to fulfill an obligation to an important duty." (Merriam-Webster, 1998). When applied to health care, this is where you must provide insurance for you and your family.

After considering these two definitions, ask yourself how do things stand? Most likely, you are reading this book because you are frustrated by managed care. My guess is that you belong to a managed care plan chosen for you by someone at work. Well, here is some more bad news. You are in a system where you are responsible for your own health care. As things stand, you and I don't have many rights or options. Here are your short-term choices:

1. Subscribe to the benefits offered by your job.

2. Get your job to offer better plans.

3. Buy private insurance.

Private policies are expensive fee-for-service plans that cover more health care, whether needed or not. However, only legislators and rich people can afford to go that route. Long-term choices are to vote for other legislators, institute socialized medicine, or do something in between. Now you see how things begin to get complicated.

AMERICANS WHO HAVE A RIGHT TO HEALTH CARE

Do Americans have any "lawful claim" to health care? Yes, but you must be disabled, over 65, or have unsupported children. The Constitution provides for five fundamental rights within the current Bill of Rights. One of these *implies* the right to health care. But only for the elderly with Medicare, and the disabled and others with Medicaid. The Bill of Rights names no specific right to health care, nor does it define coverage.

AMERICANS WHO HAVE A RESPONSIBILITY FOR HEALTH CARE

The current legislation favors employers to provide coverage for employees. This means taxes are not raised and legislators keep their jobs. However, this is where the ball gets dropped. Because your employer pays, you lose your health care choice and voice. This is why health care is cheaper. No one will demand high standards. Legislators let employers experiment with cheaper health

---

WHAT IS HEALTH INSURANCE?

Some people are more averse to risk than others. For mental comfort, some people pay others to shoulder their health concerns. If many people are willing to do this, this money can be pooled and invested. Payouts are made from the interest earned.

Are these people gambling on your health? No, because they know ages and medical histories. They have statistical programs that figure probabilities of people getting sick. Previously, everyone could get insurance easily because of the large pools. With HMOs, it has become a science. HMOs define policies tightly and access lower risk populations. Things are much more complicated.

plans on you. Expensive, fee-for-service plans are a thing of the middle class past. But are employers *providing* your health care? Indirectly, benefits are a part of your salary. Some employers give you an option. You can have a higher salary with no health benefits, or less salary and more benefits. If you pick the latter, you are paid in health care dollars.

Therefore, you have a say in how you spend your health care salary. Ask your employer how much health care costs per employee. You may be getting paid less than you think. Employers need to know your health care needs if (s)he is choosing your plan. You have more rights than you think. Especially since you are responsible for providing your own health care.

UNIVERSAL ACCESS

What about people without benefits who do not have a right to care? This concern is where rational minds differ. And there are several schools of thought. One is universal coverage, where America adopts socialized medicine. (This is addressed in Chapter 12.) Another is universal access, which is what we have today. It is the process by which all citizens are guaranteed *access* to health care. Doctors and hospitals cannot discriminate against indigents or those who cannot pay. To a large extent, hospitals and providers must care for a proportionate amount of indigent patients. However, there are loopholes to dismiss these unprofitable patients. But who ends up paying? The answer is: doctors and hospitals, and this is the reason loopholes are found. Guaranteed access does not mean guaranteed payment. Nowhere is it written that promising access means someone will pay the tab.

A FEDERAL BILL OF RIGHTS FOR HMO PATIENTS

We have seen attempts by the Clinton administration and Democrats to create an HMO patient's bill of rights. The Clintons attempted a more liberal and socialized health care reform initially. But their ideas were costly and unpopular with the

Republican Congress of the 1990s. Republicans favor big businesses and free enterprise. The theory behind managed care was to let big businesses, the health insurance industry, find a solution by rearranging responsibilities and incentives. Their reward was profits. HMOs were the brainchild of Paul Ellwood, of the Jackson Hole group (Belkin, 1996).

In theory, managed care works well. But in practice, severe compromises are expected of certain parties. Unfortunately, some compromises are life versus death. (The theory of managed care and the HMO perspective is explored in Chapter 7.)

Meanwhile, a *federal* health care bill of rights may not affect everyone. It affects federal employees, veterans, and Americans with a federal right to health care. These are the elderly Medicare patients, and government employees. Medicare patients are sold in blocks to HMOs for health care, as are government employees. These people may find themselves in unlicensed HMOs under capitated contracts.

A STATE BILL OF RIGHTS FOR HMO PATIENTS

If a bill of rights is to affect all other employees or state Medicaid patients, it must come from your state. Your state has the tools to make and enforce a state bill of health care rights. Each state has an agency that regulates managed care entities. Examples of these

---

CAPITATION

Capitation means "per person" or a set rate. It is prepaid health care, or a set fee per person per month. If the government sets capitation rates, HMOs do not need a license. The purpose of a license is to assess the ability to bear risk and set premiums. But if the government sets the premiums, unlicensed HMOs do not bear risk.

agencies are a Division of Insurance, or Department of Health. If a new HMO wants to operate in your state, it must apply to your state agency for a license to bear risk in your state. Each state has different rules and regulations that govern each HMO. And each state has its own watchdog—the insurance commissioner. This person audits and enforces your state's rules that affect managed care. This is exactly where a state bill of rights is helpful. Unfortunately, a commissioner has little power if your state has few rules and no budget. Many employees are needed to audit charters and weed out questionable practicing HMOs.

HMOs are monopolies, by definition. And monopolies are illegal. However, most states have waivers that allow and encourage HMOs to act as monopolies.

High health care costs have led states to experiment with HMOs. HMOs can relieve the higher costs of Medicaid. Some states are more progressive with HMOs than others. Nevertheless,

WHAT IS A MONOPOLY?

Monopolies are exclusive ownerships that control the supply in an industry. As HMOs merge, they control more and more health care supply. With exclusive ownership, a monopoly can set prices. HMOs fit this definition by action and appearance. (Refer to diagram on page 14.) But HMOs act strangely. While most monopolies like to raise prices, HMOs like lower prices or "premiums." It is in their best interest to attract the attention of employers and states with lower prices. Then employers and states purchase benefits. As HMOs accumulate more "covered lives," they become purchasing cooperatives. They can demand larger discounts from hospitals and providers. HMOs succeed when they control large patient markets and have price setting abilities, or when they are allowed to act as monopolies.

each state's legislative body is in the best position to regulate its managed care. Each state knows its concerns best. Therefore, states can design a better bill of rights.

The bad news is the side effects of experimentation. Some states are more conservative than others. Attempts at state waiver programs consume valuable time, money, and costly patients' rights. Much ground is lost because of continual delays, restrictions, details, and cutbacks that relate to Medicaid. Their focus is to ignore you, and find more efficient ways to deliver health care to Medicaid and Medicare patients. You are on the back burner. HMO patients are affected negatively because of Medicaid and Medicare concerns.

The good news is that costs are being contained. The working healthy will not pay as many taxes to support social health care. But the same lack of quality care felt by HMO patients now includes Medicare and Medicaid patients.

WHICH MOVE AFFECTS WHO?

A federal HMO patient's bill of rights will affect federal Medicare and government employees. If and when states set the pace, a state health care bill of rights will affect state HMOs; specifically, it will affect HMOs that cover employees and Medicare. States can regulate and enforce patients' rights closer. If both federal and state rights occur, then everyone is covered.

Of course, there are loopholes for the creative. Employers who self-insure health care for their employees are immune to a health care bill of rights. (These complexities will be discussed in Chapter 6, under ERISA.)

References
Belkin, L. (12-8-96). "But What About Quality?" *The New York Times Magazine.*
Merriam-Webster (1998). *The New Merriam-Webster Dictionary.* Merriam-Webster Publishers, Inc: Springfield, Massachusetts.

CHAPTER 3

Who Are the Players?

Things are not as they seem. Integrated health care appears to be improving health care. Everyone seems to be working together for a change. The advantage is continuity of care—connecting clinic care with hospital care and home health care—through computer networks. For example, rather than reorder lab tests in the hospital and the clinic, all areas can boot up your latest values. But appearances are deceiving. There are hidden agendas in the system that affect care negatively. And it is time for things to change. But when changes are made, it affects the whole network. An HMO patient's bill of rights is, essentially, redesigning health care. And redesigning health care is not as clear cut as you may think. A bill of rights means power is redistributed. As the cliché goes, there is strength in numbers. The group with the most power will decide how to use their power advantages against the other players.

RATIONAL BEHAVIOR

Economists define rational behavior as predicting how people will behave given changing economic motivations and conditions. When lawmakers invent financial incentives or disincentives to change the supply and demand for health care, economists sit back, watch, and predict how people will behave. So far, the following rational behavior has occurred.

▲ Co-payments and deductibles are increased. If patients must pay each time they use health care, they will not abuse their health care benefits.

- ▲ HMOs pay hospitals smaller monthly fees for more members' health care needs. In return for promises of more patients, HMOs receive larger discounts.
- ▲ If hospitals put pressure on doctors, they will keep patients out of the hospital. Then hospitals can pocket the fees.
- ▲ Doctors will ration health care, when given financial incentives or penalties. When offered bonuses or rewards, they will keep patients out of hospitals.

Now, everyone has been given reasons to use less care. But each of these motives is shortsighted. These attempts to cut costs also motivate a rational behavior—to cut corners. Currently, there are no laws against cutting corners.

WHEN ONE CHANGE AFFECTS MANY

When rules are changed, we must consider how all stakeholders will react. Rules motivate players to find loopholes. For example, high prices prevent people from buying expensive things. What happens when we get an HMO patient's bill of rights? Health care costs will go up substantially. But employers pay directly for health care. This will motivate employers to behave rationally, meaning, cut spending. Their best interests will be to avoid expensive health care benefits. Employers can hire part-time employees and pay fewer benefits. Or they can self-insure under ERISA, and make their own rules. Then, *more* people will have *less* health care. If these people become disabled or ill, they could become a burden to the state. Then there will be more government patients supported by less working people. Taxes will increase. All ramifications must be considered. We must be careful of what we ask—we may get it.

INTEGRATED HEALTH CARE NETWORKS

Picture integrated health care as a monster with three arms. The government is the brain that regulates what one arm does in relation to the other arms. Today, HMOs have the least amount of rules and the most amount of power in health care. At present, they are the dominant hand.

THE SUPPLY OF HEALTH CARE

These three arms represent the supply of health care. In order to control costs, these three arms practice some sort of rationing. (This is called supply-side rationing and will be discussed in Chapter 9.) Each arm is responsible for certain details. Here is the personality of each arm.

Hospital Systems	HMO/Insurance Companies	Medical Groups
Inpatient Services	Large Numbers of Members	Patients
Ancillary Services	Capital from Stockholders	Existing Market Presence
Outpatient Clinics	Managed Care Expertise	Organized Physician Groups
Emergency Services	Databases Identifying Cost-Efficient Providers	Leadership
Complex Tertiary Care		Primary Care Gatekeeping
Management Information Systems	Information Systems that Track Costs and Outcomes	Practice Guidelines
		Specialty Services
Health Care Education	Health Promotion	Health Care Expertise
In-home Services	Marketing/Contracting	Outpatient Clinics/ Procedures
	Government Lobbies	Less Powerful Lobbies

THE DEMAND FOR HEALTH CARE

Indirectly, the demand side for health care is the patient's. Directly, it is those who purchase health care benefits— the employers or the government.

If demand-side rationing were to occur, your employer or the state would give you dollars to spend on health care directly. The middlemen would be eliminated. In this case, you would make a budget for health care spending, track your costs, and decide what treatments purchased the best outcomes. Although this popular solution is termed medical savings accounts (MSAs), they present two major disadvantages.

- ▲ Under current laws, this money is taxable. This means MSA dollars buy less health care.
- ▲ The other concern is the return to the fee-for-service days. No middleman audits your doctors' spending. Providers can order tests you do not need and hospitals may try to keep you unnecessarily.

OTHER ECONOMIC FACTORS THAT CREATE DEMAND

- ▲ *A perceived scarcity scares consumers into wanting more health care.*
- ▲ *Decreasing health care costs enables people to afford more services.*
- ▲ *Increased availability of service allows more access.*
- ▲ *Marketing and advertising personnel or entrepreneurs promote services (i.e., nurse practitioners).*
- ▲ *There's an increase in population and/or an increase in those who develop chronic health care needs.*

Without a medical degree, it is difficult for you to know exactly how much care you need. With MSAs, the power that HMOs enjoy today would be returned to hospitals and medical groups. This is fee-for-service. We learned in the 1980s that this does not work. However, with new tax incentives and the consumerism of today, patients have more knowledge.

Currently, the HMO acts as a middleman to keep hospitals and medical groups honest. But no one is keeping the middlemen honest. An HMO patient's bill of rights is that missing piece.

CHAPTER 4

On Whose Side Are Provider Groups?

How Is Your Doctor Thinking?

Now is a difficult time to be a provider. Most doctors would rather practice medicine. They want to give you the treatment you need. But health care is a scarce resource. Now providers have been delegated the job of rationing. This is not by their choice. One major type of HMO rationing is gatekeeping. (Other types of rationing are discussed in Chapter 9.)

But, whose side is the gatekeeper on, the patient's or the HMO's? Physicians are paid agents for the managed care plan. Yet, they are advocates for the patient. Ethically, how can they be responsible to both? (Meighan, 1995).

GATEKEEPING

Each HMO patient is assigned or must choose a primary care physician from a list of conservative practitioners. Then no HMO patient can receive services unless it is cleared by this person. (S)he acts as a gate guard to let in as few patients as possible. These primary care providers are given bonuses to limit services and penalties for ordering too many. Gatekeepers have the responsibility of increasing efficiency, limiting time spent with each patient, and using specialists sparingly.

CATCH-UP ECONOMICS

Prior to managed care, physicians ran health care. But things were not perfect. As mentioned earlier, some got greedy and gave the profession a negative reputation. Eventually, the government and health plans called them on their "cost control" pretenses. The physician-in-charge era was inefficient, unregulated, and much like HMOs who have a literal free reign. Older consumers remember fee-for-service as the good old days. But runaway medicine offered neither quality nor cost containment. Just as not enough health care is wrong, so is consuming too much health care. Wasting excessive health care on some when others receive none is unethical.

We are now seeing an attempt by society to overcompensate for its previous imperfections. The problem is similar to setting a thermostat in a snowstorm during a forest fire. It is difficult to find exactly the right amount of care without over or undershooting. In playing catch-up economics, we have found another extreme. We have a favored industry—HMOs. The risks of favored industries are a lack of innovation, complacency, and no incentive to practice business ethics.

POWER SHIFTS FROM PHYSICIANS TO HMOS

The power shift from doctors to HMO CEOs shows serious attempt to control costs. This control has become too stringent. And there is no room to breathe. Are protocols written by medical or by financial personnel? Are protocols flexible? How much room for innovation or progress is built in? Where is the team approach, providers and MBAs working together to define cost-effective treatments? And by whose standards is quality defined: accountants, providers, or patients?

How have physicians lost power? We see the American Medical Association (AMA) sputtering. Questionable endorsements have made AMA members evaporate. Smaller specialty associations offer collegiality and better information. Instead of paying physicians, HMOs prefer cheaper nurse practitioners to deliver primary care. They provide the same services but cost less. (The ethics of this are discussed in Chapter 9.) Medical schools are receiving less funding and are told to produce fewer future providers. Older physicians are retiring rather than suffer through the HMOs' school of hard knocks. All these things means there are fewer physicians to ration care to the same amount of patients. For performing more work, today's physicians receive less pay. The larger salaries now go to HMO CEOs. All this paints a dismal picture for providers.

PROVIDER-SPONSORED HMOS

Physician Martin Merry refuses to give in to HMOs. On the contrary, he says, the time is now for physicians. He admits physicians played their hands poorly in the last 30 years. However, knowledge is power. And knowledge of health care is the trump card held by physicians. Managed care has one thing in its favor, and that is cost containment. But the best situation will be realized when quality is combined with cost containment. Physicians are needed to integrate quality into cost containment protocols. And who has more knowledge of the health care process? Physicians *are* protocols.

Rather than grieve or count lost money, the few physicians left will be courted again. The last 30 years are not a waste. They represent the experience or tools needed for the physician to provide competition to HMOs. Physicians could design a "central nervous" system, HMOs that offer quality at a lower cost. Physicians can be a competitive breed. As any other discipline, physicians resent being controlled by outsiders. Dr. Merry asks, who should control practice standards, physicians or the government? The answer to this question should be both. Currently, it is HMOs who are doing this.

The end of fee-for-service medicine could herald the beginning of a new era in physician leadership and influence. The past cannot be recreated nor should it be. Physicians lost the edge, but was the edge in making big bucks or bettering patient care? At present, reform has shifted to benefit big businesses rather than providers. But there is much unrest, and the thunder on the horizon is equilibrium approaching. Physician entrepreneurs are needed to run these HMOs. They can protect businesses from ignoring the human dimension.

Unfortunately, physician HMOs are at a disadvantage when competing with other HMOs. Quality care costs more. Their higher prices could be ignored by employers. Physician-sponsored HMOs must emphasize and carve out a niche by offering quality in HMOs. In recent surveys, overwhelming majorities admit more trust for an auto repair shop or the federal government than an HMO. Physicians are still trusted by their patients. And it is through providers that things can improve.

PHYSICIAN-SPONSORED HOSPITALS

The business of successful medicine is difficult in today's managed competition. The advantage to having physicians as managers is that quality receives a higher priority than the bottom line.

The Mayo Clinic in Rochester, Minnesota is a not-for-profit foundation that is managed by physicians. Physicians work closely with hospital administrators. Both are encouraged to be creative, sensitive, and to work with each other in crises and tension. The disadvantages are the slowed momentum and difficulty of team consensus. Here, success is felt where all understand organization dynamics, relinquish power and control, and share an understanding of health care and business competence. Another disadvantage is a separation from peers. Physicians in practice have little trust or respect for physicians in management.

In medicine, the doctor acts as an agent to provide best possible patient care because of greater knowledge. But the health care business must still deliver medicine. And medical and business ethics are difficult to separate. Medical leadership prevents exploiting patients for profit. Perhaps this is the reason Mayo has a worldwide reputation for quality.

CONCEPTUAL FLAWS

Even with prudent rationing, patients' needs must be acknowledged. If ignored, things will go wrong. The extreme is that patients may begin to panic. When third parties pay for health care, this inflates patient demand. We learned that patients can have higher expectations when health care is free. Emergency room (ER) abuse for routine problems was given as an example. Gatekeeping causes ER abuse.

Panic and fear surface when everyone must fight to get their fair share. When the food runs out, appetites grow despite full bellies. And people who are told no might be tempted to behave in irrational or unpredictable ways. These are motivations for patients to behave negatively. Too much rationing too quickly makes patients behave negatively. It is no surprise that the number of patient complaints is growing.

Provider-sponsored HMOs and hospitals may regain patients' trust. If patients were treated as responsible, mature adults, they will behave as such. Certainly, patients can be taught to use scarce resources wisely. In fact, patients should have some responsibility for costs. They may even self-ration. (This option is discussion further in Chapter 12 under MSAs.)

Currently, humans are "covered lives" that represent potential profits. Although customer service is a business term, physicians have a similar concept called bedside manner. However, there is the dilemma in improving customer service in health care. It is not clear who is the customer. Employers, not patients, choose health plans. When patients are out of the loop, we can expect customer service and beside manner to suffer.

When physicians have contracts with HMOs, are not the HMOs their customers? When HMOs sign providers' paychecks, patients' concerns are secondary to HMOs' concerns. After all, the patient is not directly allowed in on these service contracts. Physicians are being asked to serve two masters. On the one hand, doctors are expected to provide a wide variety of services, recommend the best treatments, and improve quality of life. On the other hand, they are expected to keep expenses to a minimum. Physicians must choose between the best interest of their patients and their own economic survival. When managed care enters a community, physicians are forced to work for HMOs or be left without patients. In addition, there is no guarantee for contracts to be renewed. If a provider prescribes too many services, (s)he may be left without a job. Today it is difficult to move and start over. If a physician is dismissed from another plan, s(he) may be considered unemployable (Kassirer, 1995). There are too many things wrong with this picture.

In the Hippocratic oath, physicians pledge to provide care, not restrict it.

ACCOUNTABILITY

What happens to the providers who take a stand? Physicians who keep patients in the hospital longer than allowed are penalized financially. Physicians' spending habits are tracked, compared, and profiled. This is called economic credentialing or physician profiling. Physicians who spend less per patient are the most desirable. HMOs will discriminate against physicians who practice inefficiently.

Peer review is another method to track practice patterns. Groups of doctors scrutinize individual physicians' practices. This is a way specialists can monitor each other's spending habits.

Managed care has complicated these issues further by issuing incentives and disincentives. Physicians cannot practice medical ethics with the threat of job loss. In a tightly managed care system, physicians cannot provide service that they should, cannot be patient advocates, and cannot challenge rules governing appropriate services.

ADDED COMPLEXITIES

Physicians must keep up with paperwork, and stay abreast of membership changes and new rulings when already short of time. This forces them to sign on healthier patients who are less prone to illness. This is called "cherry picking" patients. What happens when everyone fights for healthier patients? Further discrimination occurs against chronically ill patients. What happens to naive providers who allow HMOs to sign on patients who are very, very ill?

Physicians have further constraints on their time when they must educate patients about benefit limits. Who else can explain what services patients are and are not entitled? Then physicians must listen to upset patients blame and chastise them for the loss of their benefits. Since employers switch plans on their employees every two to three years, this becomes a full-time scramble.

If physicians are too busy for patient care already, consider the following situations. Legally, a physician is accountable for every harmful patient limit in their contracts. Negligence is illegal, punishable with large monetary rewards for injured parties. Moreover, physicians are accountable for other physicians' behaviors in their provider group. The burden of malpractice is shared among partners, and is also punishable by large sums. Today's physician needs a law degree to successfully practice within the managed care model. The HMOs have provisions so they cannot be sued.

COOPERATIVE CARE

Here is a potential solution to managing chronically ill patients in HMOs. When confronted with a continually increasing patient load, one doctor found a way out. Rather than leveraging quality for efficiency, Dr. John Scott works smarter, not harder. Other colleagues agreed that substandard care was endangering the well-being of their patients. So these Kaiser doctors hold support groups to provide comfort and teaching to every clinic patient.

> ## HOW LITIGATION TAKES MEDICINE A STEP BACKWARD
>
> *"...[how can we] change from just looking for the bad apples."*
> —D. Berwick
>
> *Mistakes and litigation have a cause and effect relationship. Lawsuits prevent health professionals from sharing information when things go wrong. A fear has been created that focusing on errors emphasizes human weakness. But the finger that points to blame also points to opportunity. Medical mistakes should represent a drawing board. Improved performance and ideas can only come from spotlighting and studying deficiencies. How can we foster creativity or innovation with tight practice guidelines in a legal environment that punishes honesty?*

The result is "giant doctor's office visits" or Cooperative Care Clinics. Co-op care targets groups of chronically ill patients with diseases such as diabetes, arthritis, hypertension, and heart disease. Rather than one patient at a time, this provides group chronic care. Quality teaching is provided at reduced costs.

This is a long-term solution to managing the high-risk patients who require costly care. Monthly support group meetings are taught by physicians, nurses, pharmacists, and dieticians about treatments, tests, medications, diet, and exercise specific to the shared illness. During the meetings, nurses check blood pressure or blood sugar as they would for a clinic visit. Charts may be browsed by patients and their caregivers to stimulate questions about their care. Flu or pneumonia vaccines are offered. This conglomerated distribution of information saves private repetition in clinic visits, thus allowing personal attention to be devoted to individual physical exams. Serendipitously, efficiency has not been the only positive outcome. Grant monies from various foundations are arriving to proliferate this answer to the chronic care question. However, patients' responses have created the greatest impact. The "experts" of chronic disease are providing strength *to each other*, sometimes overlooked in the traditional doctor's office model, for free. Coping with loss of independence or dignity, loneliness, and aging are conditions that a physician cannot treat.

ADVANTAGES OF COOPERATIVE CARE

Previously, the long-term piece was missing in the cost containment puzzle. Today's healthy young HMO members are tomorrow's aging population. This is the perfect solution for capitation in the Medicare and Medicaid populations. Projected figures on caring for chronic illness coupled with aging populations are sobering. There are few other suggestions. How else can standards be maintained, patients' needs addressed, and gatekeeping occur for the chronically ill? Is mass medical care the answer?

Pilot studies show less utilization of health care by co-op patients over time.

CO-OP PATIENTS' UTILIZATION OVER ONE YEAR
(Lumsdon, 1995)

ER Visits	Down 39%
Hospital Admissions	Down 24%
Length of Hospital Stays	Down 20%

In addition, computer software has been developed to alert case managers when members are having trouble at home or have other unmet needs. Perhaps this idea is not so new. Support groups and group therapy have been around for a while. However, this is a new take on support groups. New goals for new groups with specific outcomes has powerful potential. Extrapolation to other conditions such as HIV, Alzheimer's, cancer, transplant patients, and any "chronic" illness can be attempted in this model. So, too, might *temporary* chronic states such as pregnancy, or alcohol and drug addictions be addressed.

DISADVANTAGES

The idea provokes many questions. For example, persons inhibited by public speaking are penalized critical discussion time with their provider. What about non-compliant patients? Will they require special teaching and therefore special charging? Ethically, can HMOs mandate doctors to practice collective medicine? And how will those who practice collective medicine successfully be rewarded versus those who are unsuccessful?

The present methods of managing chronic care are certainly not perfect, nor is this alternative without its flaws. This trend's promise of better care at lower prices deserves a second, but cautious look. Further investments of time, energy, and money are required to provide stronger evidence of goal achievement. Even more convincing would be *less* utilization of time, energy, and money with better outcomes. The ultimate success will be determined in how an HMO enforces participation, or more important, measures *learning*.

Legislation allows providers to form their own regulated HMOs. Previously, this had been prevented by antitrust legislation. But since managed care is a monopoly, physician HMOs offer options for patients with choices an opportunity to vote with their feet. Things could change drastically. Physicians have been given the power to compete by offering quality. This will force HMOs to offer quality in their plans. By allowing competition for patients, quality would improve and costs would remain competitive. Or at least it would all be less volatile.

This will help HMO patients get better care and have more rights.

References

Berwick, D. (1-5-89). "Continuous Improvement as an Ideal in Healthcare." *NEJM 320,* (1), 53–56.

Gatty, B. (11-1-96). "Ensuring Quality of Care Proves Elusive." *Physician Management.*

Kassierer, J. (7-6-95). "Managed Care and the Morality of the Marketplace." *NEJM.*

Lumsdon, K. (11-5-95). "Working Smarter, not Harder." *Hospitals & Health Networks.*

Marren, J. & Hynes, D. (7-1-95). "Legal Issues in Accepting Capitation." *Physician Executive.*

Meighan, S. (1995). "Where Have All the Primary Care Physicians Gone?" A Socratic discourse. *Health Care Management Review 20,* (3), 64–67.

Merry, Martin (9-1-96). "The Time Is Now." *Physician Executive 22,* (6), 4–17.

CHAPTER 5

On Whose Side Is the Hospital System?

How Are Treatment Centers Thinking?

"The ten thousand things carry Yin and embrace Yang. They achieve harmony by combining these forces. For one gains by losing and loses by gaining."
—Tao Te Ching

Now is a difficult time to be a hospital. Many of the hospitals who supported the indigent or patients who could not pay have closed. Yet the technological age requires each competitive hospital to have expensive MRI and CT machines occupying square footage in their radiology departments. Meanwhile, complete face-lifts for computer integration are required for updating to electronic patient records. Some facilities have chosen to eliminate services, such as obstetrics. Why? Providing "luxury" services such as delivering babies in low birth rate areas is not cost effective. Focusing on needs of the community is one way to stay alive. When backed in financial corners, hospitals have closed wings, made cutbacks, layoffs, or salary decreases. These options are mere Band-Aids to *hide* the bleeding. Drastic times have required more drastic measures.

HOSPITAL NETWORKS

Hospital response to managed care has been to form megahospital systems. The power afforded to these networks is challenging the power of managed care organizations (MCOs). MCOs reign by virtue of their size and, therefore, power. When HMOs collect

> ## IS TECHNOLOGY THE CAUSE FOR RISING COSTS?
>
> *At what point does our ability to generate medical advances outrun our desire to pay for them? We spend more health care dollars per person than any other country. The same is true of technology dollars. We spend more per person on computers, faxes, and phones than any other country. But there is no cost containment on technology.*
>
> *Health care insurance is the reason we demand medical advances. If patients are "not paying" for benefits, why shouldn't we want more? If health care is free, there is no incentive for consumers to contain costs. Health benefits provided by others induces excessive spending (Newhouse, 1993).*

huge numbers of patients, they become a coveted customer to hospitals. Whoever has patients, has power. Hospitals and provider groups must court these HMOs for the right to care for their patients. Because MCOs are so strong, they can demand reasonable discounts. Sometimes these discounts are unreasonable. In return, hospitals have guaranteed patients for the life of a contract. Every year or two, contracting and discount negotiation starts again. When hospitals are desperate for patients, they agree to cutthroat contracts rather than allow the HMO to take its patients to their competitor. This has caused many hospitals to dissolve or be bought out by hospital giants.

Hospitals that make this choice are known to have "sold their souls." When a hospital must operate for a profit, the focus changes from saving lives to making money. Stockholders come before patients. When stock is sold to shareholders, so is decision-making. Voters want big dividends, large profit margins, and leaders who can create dollar signs. Research money vaporizes and patient progress is forgotten.

ADVANTAGES OF HOSPITAL NETWORKS

There is a positive side to hospitals as systems. They can act as collusive groups to counter HMO demands. In addition, networks can better control other costs. One set of administrators in a network can set contracting "policies" for many hospitals. This sets a united front. It is the only recourse hospitals can use to act as monopolies. Hospitals as larger systems can take their turn to demand discounts from computer vendors and suppliers. Even not-for-profit hospitals are finding protection in numbers. Unlikely partnering is occurring between previous enemies. Hospitals run by Catholic, Methodist, and Lutheran denominations are seeing eye to eye for the first time. But in the scramble for marriages, patients are left out.

CONCEPTUAL FLAWS

Managed care is not consumer-driven because patients are excluded in hospital services, contracting, and coverage decisions. Most purchasers of health plans are employers. They lean toward cheaper plans that offer fewest frills. If patients do not have choices, cost, not quality, dominates decisions. Hospitals are forced to change their perspectives from quality-focused to cost-focused in order to compete. Hospitals are trying to please HMOs and employers, not patients. They are attracted to quantity discounts, not quality care. Therefore, you can expect hospital services to get worse. Hospitals and physicians in a capitated system:

- ▲ may not provide all the services they should,
- ▲ may not always be patient advocates, and
- ▲ may be reluctant to challenge the rules governing which services are appropriate.

In some cases, contracts forbid hospitals and physicians to disclose the existence of services not covered by a plan. Hospitals have no choice but to fight over precious contracts with HMOs. Without patient input, there is further potential for collusion among MCOs and hospitals to offer even fewer services.

A DIFFERENT MISSION: RESEARCH AND EDUCATION

Hospitals try to contract with health plans that:

- ▲ recruit the healthiest patients,
- ▲ exclude the chronically ill,
- ▲ ration by making care inconvenient to obtain, and
- ▲ deny care in the name of profit.

Where do missions of research, education, and supporting the indigent fit in a managed care world? Managed care has squeezed most hospitals to the point of reducing or eliminating research or education. The University Hospital networks are the only ones left attempting this mission. But academic institutions must compete with hospital networks who are more efficient. As a result, these facilities are losing money. These institutions have little choice but to ask the government for subsidies. Taxes must support non-profit institutions with different missions. Why aren't for-profit hospitals with growing bottom lines doing research? Because there are no profits. Comparing hospitals with different missions is like comparing apples with oranges. Academic costs are not felt by for-profit hospitals. Academic facilities cannot lower prices or grant huge discounts. The demise of the University Hospital is inevitable under this system. The rules are not fair. Competition by costs does not factor in creating progress. This inequity could lead to extinction of future knowledge.

SCARCE HEALTH CARE RESOURCES

Health care is a scarce resource when demand for health care outweighs supply. Either the supply-side or the demand-side of health care will be asked to economize. Since it is difficult to control demand, present government regulation favors and motivates changes in the supply-side. Managed care does a fabulous job. It cuts costs while making profits. This relieves the government of direct rationing and periodic review of rationing mechanisms. Network profits from hospitals and HMOs can be taxed. In theory, this money is used to support Medicare, Medicaid, and other social programs without additional taxes. Wealth is encouraged, made, and redistributed. This is the reason for delays in a patient's bill of rights. To the government bureaucrats, this system is not broken. So why fix it? Health care is held in bondage to big business. If legislators are slaves of HMOs, so are hospitals and other stakeholders.

SCARCE HUMAN RESOURCES

Using this logic, where and how can the scales of justice balance? What is fair use of health care? Which is more important, healthy profits or healthy taxpayers? And when do people change from being patients to economic units? Each human is a unique organism. His or her creativity will never grace the universe again. The ingenuity of these living, breathing entities are also a scarce resource.

One health care network chose to suffer the loss of a large contract in order to maintain higher patient standards. Defining one's principles over economic considerations is a lesson for all involved in health care. Pinon Management, based in Lakewood, Colorado, is reaffirming personal and organizational philosophies. Entities should learn a lesson from Pinon's absolutes in quality care standards.

BALANCING YIN AND YANG

Jeff Jerebker, of Pinon, shares how quality of life in a long-term care facility cannot conflict with the bottom line. Being of equal importance, one cannot exist without the other. Pinon refused to leverage quality by the overextension of liabilities, when the end result would be patient exploitation. Returns must be reasonable for the circumstances. And quality of life demands must not be wasteful. Therein lie the keys to success.

When nuns ran hospitals, no one worried about costs. Their faith told them that the Lord would provide. Now, hospitals are for-profit entities. Shareholders want their cut. Health-related employees focus on costs and not profit. This is a 180-degree shift. We must not let the pendulum that cuts wasteful spending endanger basic medicine. Although a long-term care facility, Pinon has drawn their line. Other health care institutions, too, must balance cutbacks and standards.

The delivery of health care is a unique challenge revolving around the human dimension. Human life is to be respected. It does not represent a commodity on which to take risks for earning unreasonably high returns. Investors with superior earning demands want dividends at the expense of quality of life. Our society should be encouraging these investors to look elsewhere. More realistic profit expectations are found in markets such as shopping centers, warehouses, or real estate. How will this happen when health care remains for-profit? Are the gains for some worth the losses by others? Perhaps our society is losing its balance in regarding the value of human life.

Who, then, is America to sit in judgment of the lack of human rights in other countries?

References

Jerebker, Jeff (1997). *Pinon News: A Long-Term Care Journal 6*, (1), 1–2.

Newhouse, J. (1993). "An Iconoclastic View of Healthcare Cost Containment." *Health Affairs 12*, 152–171.

CHAPTER 6

On Whose Side Is Your State?

On Whose Side Is Your Employer?

What do states and employers have in common? Both need HMOs to provide health care for their employees or poverty patients. Therefore, in certain conditions, states and employers have the same point of view. And their perspective as stakeholders might be seen and used interchangeably. They both share concerns for the costs of health care. Both want easy yet inexpensive access for their wards. They, in effect, are major patrons or customers of health care.

WHO ELSE PAYS FOR HEALTH CARE SERVICES

▲ The U.S. taxpayers who fund Medicare and Medicaid
▲ Employers, unions, universities, and others who provide group plans
▲ Privately funded insurers or indemnity plans
▲ Malpractice lawsuits of companies and corporation, such as tobacco and implant manufacturers

Therefore, these are the folks who drive the health care economy.

STATE INNOVATIONS

For true HMO patient rights reform, watch the states. States are in the best position to make and enforce health care standards. Federal health care reform has silently shifted to the states in the form of managed care restructuring (Lutz, 1995). HMOs are now willing to take on billion dollar programs with state and federal approval. The federal government, through HCFA, has granted waivers from antitrust to most states to operate managed care Medicaid and Medicaid programs. Federal permission or waivers allow states to:

- ▲ design their own eligibility rules,
- ▲ expand coverage to enroll the uninsured, and
- ▲ require enrollees to stay with a plan for more than six months.

With managed care, states hope to reduce health care spending while expanding access to greater, more uninsured residents. States will sell poverty patients to HMOs for care. Through HMOs, primary care physicians will gatekeep. This will eliminate the costly trend of ER visits for HMO and government patients.

WHO IS HCFA (HEALTH CARE FINANCING ADMINISTRATION)?

HCFA is an administrative agency established by the federal government to regulate seniors' Medicare benefits. It also deals with state Medicaid issues. Although states run Medicaid, federal funds match state funds spent on poverty patient care. If a federal HMO patient's bill of rights occurs, it will be regulated by HCFA.

Here are a few of the controversial concepts that various states are exploring:

▲ health care vouchers or credit cards with spending limits,

▲ funding to states that have more poverty patients, such as New York and California, and

▲ access to the working uninsured only.

HOW MUCH IS TOO MUCH?

Cutting costs is a double-edged sword. States need to worry about putting their own providers and hospitals out of business. Implications to cut health care costs mean less inpatient business. Less inpatient business threatens hospital closures because of revenue losses. Previously, this revenue was used to pay operating costs. Some capped payment rates do not meet actual operating costs for increasing health care demands.

LEGISLATORS' INTERESTS

A state bill of rights would be simple. States have regulatory agencies that could enforce HMO standards. But if consumer groups force a bill of rights to come to vote, will the legislators listen? Legislators must worry about the costs they inflict on HMOs. ERISA prevents some of the damage (see box on page 47). And HMO lobbyists have much power. HMOs can raise money by selling more stocks. This is money that supports legislative campaigns. But present health care delivery is losing the trust of the people it cares for—patients who vote. Legislators are torn between voters and campaign support. Money needed for campaign support is a higher priority than voters' needs. Notoriety must come first, before winning voters. If campaign contributors are alienated, a campaign cannot last until an election.

ERISA

ERISA is the Employee Retirement Income Security Act of 1974. Under ERISA, some employers do not have to follow state rules that regulate employees' health care benefits.

This rule was thought to encourage more employers to offer health care benefits. It is a safeguard that tries not to penalize employers for providing at least a few health benefits.

Sometimes it is cheaper for employers to self-insure rather than pay an HMO. Employers may hire a Third Party Administer (TPA) to coordinate their employees' health benefits. But this TPA could be an HMO or act as a managed care entity. This means employees may belong to HMOs under a TPA. In this case, they are immune to a state HMO patient's bill of rights under ERISA.

ERISA would need to be changed. If not, there will be a scramble for all employers to self-insure health benefits for their employees and to avoid the higher costs of quality (Mashaw, 1994).

CONCEPTUAL FLAWS

Here are other reasons why things have become so complicated.

- ▲ Standards in health care will raise prices. Why would states want to raise the prices they pay for health care? These folks do not want to see a health care bill of rights. They want the opposite—less rights that mean lower prices for their poverty patients. This represents a large majority of people who could get more health care. Also, it is counterintuitive for taxpayers to want higher taxes.
- ▲ A bill of rights will not improve customer service. Your state or your employer contracts with HMOs. Customer

service is not their concern. It is the problem of your hospital or provider group. HMOs, the states, and your employer want to give you less. Who is the state, but your legislators. They will be swayed by whomever offers them a sweeter deal. Employers hire big business lobbyists who support their party and campaigns. This represents their job. Until voters unite, this represents a stronger and more organized voice. Personally, most legislators are not affected by low-standard health care. Most likely, they buy VIP insurance or fee-for-service health care. With a bill of rights, expect customer service to patients to get worse.

▲ A health care bill of rights does not solve the problem of moral hazard, but encourages it.

▲ The HMO patient's bill of rights will increase health care costs for everyone. This means tax hikes. Legislators don't want the blame for higher taxes. This motivates legislative foot dragging, a very rational behavior in their position.

MORAL HAZARD

Moral hazard is the label economists give abusing health care due to insurance. Simply stated, when something is purchased by others for your use, it is considered "free." This encourages everyone to become complacent about costs. But when you must pay for something yourself, you are much more conscious of costs. Health care becomes expensive to you when you must make responsible decisions for consumption. You may even use less of it. Meanwhile, you and others will continue to consume more of it without considering the effects of your behavior. Health care benefits paid by others leads to inflated patient demand.

▲ When patients' demands are not heard, again, panic mounts to unreasonable levels. Patients sue at lower thresholds. Unfortunately, legislators are responding with proposals for litigation caps for state and federal hospitals. Currently, some HMOs are immune to lawsuits. Look at your policy—you may find the words "mandatory" and "binding arbitration." This means, malpractice claims and other disputes are resolved by a panel of arbitrators. But when arbitrators are hired, the HMO signs their check. Arbitrators may not be rehired if they find an HMO at fault. This encourages recklessness. Without accountability, the standard of health care drops. Who really wins?

▲ HMOs are not the bad guys. They are playing by the rules made for them by legislators. HMOs can afford to cut more services to be even more efficient. Quality is not a driving factor for patients. State legislators and

---

SHOULD YOU SUE YOUR HMO?

Employers may be held responsible in their HMO's malpractice litigation. The more HMOs are sued, the more it undermines voluntary, employer-provided health care insurance. This could add millions to the ranks of the uninsured.

Remember ERISA, which encourages well-intentioned employers to self-insure health insurance? Because of ERISA, some have health care benefits where otherwise they would have none. If HMOs pass punitive costs on to employers, they will forego offering benefits.

Suing an HMO could come back to haunt you when your employer drops your health care coverage. If you plan to sue an HMO for punitive damages, make sure it is enough to buy health care insurance for a long time.

employers encourage this by continuing to choose low-cost HMOs. HMOs have brought costs down; therefore states and employers are happy using HMOs to ration your health care.

ONE STATE'S SOLUTION

States sell groups of welfare patients to HMOs to coordinate health care. This means the large welfare population joins the HMO patient fight for health care rights. We know the cost for quality health care for welfare patients will be felt in higher taxes. Or will it?

Today's trend is for states to limit single parents on welfare benefits for two years. During that time, money, training for employment, child care, medical benefits, and help to find employment will be provided. If employers cover health care costs, then, eventually, taxes will go down. Wisconsin's overhaul of welfare and Medicaid has resulted in a 60 percent spending decrease in the last decade. How? They constructed assistance around a job and not a check.

Does this discriminate against blacks, women, and children? Does this encourage crime, drugs, and prostitution because "women gotta do what they gotta do"? Not necessarily—there are rewards in providing for oneself and family. These programs offer child and health care to previous welfare recipients, and have created thousands of jobs. Jobs that lead to health care benefits.

CONCEPTUAL FLAWS

There are many problems with this system. Hiring agencies are paid to find jobs for workers similar to HMOs. People are being forced to work against their will. This creates an incentive to show up drunk for interviews, so as not to be hired. Hiring agencies are prepaid to find jobs for workers just as HMOs are prepaying for health care chargees. A fixed payment is made to serve xxx amounts of families. The faster people are employed and off entitlement, the more money the agencies make. Is money saved when it is merely redirected? Is this a permanent idea or will the subsidies diminish? Why are mothers required to work and not fathers of children on assistance? Is Wisconsin redirecting welfare traffic to other states? Are there increased applicants for welfare and Medicaid in other states? These questions have not yet been answered.

FOR YOU TO GET RIGHTS, YOU WILL PAY MORE THAN YOUR SHARE

Overall population is declining. Less childbearing women means less potential welfare numbers. How much of Wisconsin's 60 percent decrease is explained by this? And Wisconsin's success cannot be extrapolated to areas such as New York and California. Clearly, these populations are different. Imagine the costs of patients' rights when all states' poverty groups belong to HMOs.

There is a point to this. It is an attempt to describe the magnitude that an HMO bill of rights will cost. When rights for Medicaid patients are included this means higher state taxes. To ask HMOs or employers to shell out the costs for more health care is upsetting a delicate balance. HMOs will declare bankruptcy. Employers will not provide benefits. What then, socialized medicine?

Again, we need to be mindful for what we are asking. In whatever form the bill of rights takes, all-inclusive or not, pain will be felt in higher costs. How much are you willing to pay in higher taxes for an HMO patient's bill of rights that includes more health care for Medicaid and Medicare patients?

CONCLUSION

A compromise must be made somewhere. Either the tax laws must change to support medical savings accounts or HMOs must offer quality and patients' choice. A bill of rights is a vehicle of change, although an expensive one.

The most economically efficient method would be to give patients the tools to reward the best providers—freedom of choice. States and employers do not give consumers these tools nor any responsibility for health care costs. Therefore, there is no reason for consumers to limit health care use.

References

DeParle, Jason (8-24-97). "Getting Opal Caples to Work." *The New York Times Magazine.*

Lutz, S. (1-23-95). "For Real Reform, Watch the States." *Modern Healthcare.*

Mashaw, J. (Winter, 93–94). "Taking Federalism Seriously: The Case for State Led Healthcare Reform." *Domestic Affairs.*

Zaldivar, R. (9-25-97). "HMO Standards Outlined." *The Denver Post.*

On Whose Side Is Your HMO or Other Managed Care Organization?

CHAPTER 7

Prospective payments for health care is not new. In 1888, the Sisters of St. Francis in Chippewa Falls, Wisconsin sold $5 tickets to lumberjacks for one year of health care benefits. These passes covered:

- ▲ all medical and surgical treatment,
- ▲ free baths,
- ▲ care at any affiliated Wisconsin or U.S. hospital, and
- ▲ on-site or mail order prescriptions.

These nurse-nuns netted $20,000 the first year, enough to build a modern hospital. This hospital grew into the St. Joseph network. Why did it work for the nuns? It worked because they used competition based on quality. And they were a not-for-profit system that returned profits to the hospital. Their *true* focus was on community wellness. Today's managed care is for-profit. These corporations must return most of the profits to stockholders in the form of dividends, and less money goes to patient care.

ECONOMIES OF SCALE

What is the theory of managed care? It is not the same as in the days of the nuns. Today's managed care is more complicated. It involved integrated delivery systems and computerized networks. Integrated delivery networks are physicians, hospital, and insurers who work to improve the health of its enrolled population.

THE BIRTH OF MANAGED CARE (CHA & CMCC)

WORKINGMEN ATTENTION

Protect yourself by buying a ticket on St. Joseph's Hospital, Chippewa Falls, Wisconsin.

This hospital is located on Stanley hill, corner of Spruce and Pear streets; the above cut is a good illustration of the building, with the new addition, which is one of the finest hospitals in the northwest, with all the latest modern improvements. Electric bells in the rooms; the building is lighted by gas and heated by steam and hot water throughout; each story contains a large bathroom.

Tickets bought on this hospital are good on a large number of other Sisters' hospitals located in the principal cities of Wisconsin and other states.

St. Joseph's, Chippewa Falls; St. John's, Springfield, Ill.; Sacred Heart Hospital, Eau Claire; St. Elizabeth's hospital, Belleville, Ill.; St. Mary's Hospital, Decatur, Ill.; St. Vincent's hospital, Green Bay, Wis.; St. Joseph's, Highland, Ill.; St. Anthony's hospital, Effingham, Ill.; St. Mary's hospital, East St. Louis; St. Clara's hospital, Lincoln, Ill.; St Francis hospital, Lichfield, Ill.; St Mary's Hospital, Streater, Ill.; St Joseph's hospital, St. Charles, Mo.; St. Nicholas hospital, Sheboygan, Wis. Seven dollars and a half ($7.50) tickets are issued, good for one year.

You are entitled to medicine at the hospital dispensary at Chippewa Falls, or it will be sent free to any part of the country if you send the number of your ticket.

For medicine always address St. Joseph's hospital, Chippewa Falls, and state in plain writing your own address and nearest post office and express office. While in camp have your order endorsed by your foreman.

The best local physicians are connected with these hospitals.

Lumbermen, remember that our ticket is worth all that it promises. There is no danger either that it becomes worthless thru bankruptcy, which has happened with other companies selling tickets. No other company or corporation has a right to claim that their tickets are good on the St. Joseph's hospital. Beware of misrepresentations by outside agents.

While we do not bribe logging firms for the exclusive right of selling tickets in their camps, we ask for ourselves the privilege of selling in all camps, to give the workingmen the benefit of a free choice. All we ask for is fair competition. Every agent has his territory, and consequently, there will be but one agent in each camp.

Logging firms will please never cash an order of ours unless endorsed by the Sister Superior of St. Joseph's hospital.

Essentially, it is prepaid health care. In return for a per person dollar amount, enrollees receive seamless care. Seamless care is care from clinic to hospital to home health to nursing home or hospice. All have computerized integration and knowledge of your working patient records. These new incentives introduce economies of scale to reduce duplication, coordinate services across settings, and ensure that enrollees receive care in appropriate and cost-effective settings. It is a way to be more efficient and provide health care at a lower cost.

Integrated managed care works in three ways.

- ▲ There is an intended focus on community wellness. Through prevention, all providers within the network improve the health of the community. The goal is to keep you healthy, and out of the system, rather than wait and give you health care advice when you are sick.

- ▲ There is a coordinated continuum of care from clinic to hospital to home health care. Patients are treated in the most appropriate and least costly settings at the right time—not too much care, but the right amount in the appropriate setting.

- ▲ Economic incentives are aligned. Employers/states pay HMOs for health care benefits for their members. In turn, HMOs make capitation payments to hospitals and physicians. Each makes its own decisions about how to allocate payments among participants in the network. The provides the opportunity to negotiate price discounts, streamline administration, and increase efficiency.

MANAGED COMPETITION

Managed care is sometimes called managed competition. They are not the same thing. Since modern HMOs must act as monopolies to set prices, and since patients do not drive the economy, there is not a true "competition."

CONCEPTUAL FLAWS

In practice, there are many conflicting financial incentives and clinical demands. What appears to be a problem with managed care is actually a problem with medicine. Doctors don't know the best way to treat most illnesses. As a result, the quality and cost of

---

KINDS OF MANAGED CARE ORGANIZATIONS

The simplest way to classify HMOs is the more health care you want, the more you pay.

- ▲ IPAs or Independent Practice Associations: networks of physicians and specialists
- ▲ PHOs or Physician-Hospital Organizations: physician groups and hospitals
- ▲ Staff Model HMOs: few physicians in limited locations that are salaried HMO employees
- ▲ Group Model HMOs: more physician and specialists that contract with HMOs
- ▲ Network or mixed model HMOs: offer more convenience, coverage, and locations
- ▲ POS or Point of Service Plans: you pay to have more choices. This is fee-for-service within a managed care model.
- ▲ PPO or Preferred Provider Organizations: a POS with more restrictions
- ▲ EPO or Exclusive Provider Organization: limited choice of providers

medical procedures vary from doctor to doctor, and from region to region. And managed care, a bureaucracy accountable to nobody, has decided to exploit the variation in how doctors work (O'Reilly, 1998). This will continue as long as there are no established protocols for diagnoses.

In capitation, providers become responsible for a group of people. But there is a penalty for ordering services. And here is where greed steps in.

Employees are a group or population to be served. Employers sell employees and their families to HMOs as "covered lives." However, employees are relatively healthy patients. Obviously, they are young and energetic enough to work. Statistically, they are low-risk because they use fewer services. These employee groups represent a huge source of profit. HMOs may negotiate lower payments to providers/hospitals when they can prove they have younger, healthier members. When fewer services are used, then profits may be kept. Employees are the most appealing population to HMOs and their networks.

CHRONIC ILLNESS

What if you have a chronic illness? Or what if you use more health care? What if you are high-risk for certain genetic diseases? This becomes a problem. Here are ways to discriminate against high-risk consumers of health care:

- ▲ Neglecting to enroll you if you have a poor medical history
- ▲ Not covering preexisting illnesses
- ▲ Contracting in affluent neighborhoods where physicians serve affluent patients
- ▲ Marketing to employers only
- ▲ Neglecting to hire specialists who treat expensive illnesses such as cancer or HIV

FINANCIAL DISINCENTIVES

Each arm within a network must remain "efficient" to keep revenues higher than their expenses. But a problem occurs when each arm defines "efficient" in their own terms. HMOs ask providers to be efficient by sharing some of the risk. This means providers must reduce the number of tests and procedures down to a minimum. If they prescribe too many, they are penalized. If they prescribe too little, they are rewarded. In this way, providers are motivated to share the cost and risk for services. Their prescribing habits are monitored and profiled. And they will be held accountable. Providers that use too many services over time must be terminated. Providers that use too few services are rewarded with longer contracts.

The best way to help HMO providers to provide too few services is to have healthy HMO members. This means using employees as covered lives, only.

BOUNTY HUNTING

The *LA Times* (2-1-97) reports California HMOs use marketing techniques to obtain preferred members. HMOs pay physicians a bounty of $25 for each healthy life they direct to their HMO. There are implications to these allegations.

▲ HMOs have economic priorities. The more members HMOs have, the more power they have over other HMOs. If they have more members they get better discounts when purchasing provider and hospital services. What if HMOs can promise hospitals healthier members who need little inpatient care? This marketing and negotiation tool for lower rates attracts the attention of hospitals. They are willing to provide services for lower rates. When HMOs get huge discounts, your employers pay less for health care benefits. Low prices allow more HMOs to pick up more members and more power. The challenge for HMOs is to find healthy patients who use little health care. Why shouldn't HMOs pay doctors to hand pick these patients for them? Who else knows who and where the healthy patients are? Why wouldn't patients become commodities to be bought and sold? HMOs are for-profit entities with a responsibility to make money for their stockholders. Under current law, this is rational, legal, and the *encouraged* behavior.

▲ When HMOs must compete, advertising budgets grow. There is a temptation to spend more money on marketing and less on patient care.

▲ Business ethics and medical ethics are separate, and hybrid HMOs are held to neither. HMOs are an unregulated industry that may be a business or a medical industry. HMOs can use whichever industry's argument fits a given situation. HMOs can waver on their use of business or medical ethics.

▲ Patients trust doctors because of their knowledge. The misuse of this knowledge to direct patients toward HMOs is a breach of confidentiality. But today's doctors are employees of HMOs. Why shouldn't they react rationally to offers of positive economical benefits? If patients have a choice of plans, doctors can be paid to channel the healthy toward more generous HMOs. But how are patients to know their best choices for health care if given tainted guidance? How can doctors be trusted? What, if any, remaining freedom do patients have in health care decisions?

WHO PAYS FOR CLINICAL TRIALS?

HMOs will not cover the cost of inefficient or experimental treatments and procedures. They do not create profits. Why should HMOs pay for expensive treatments based on a few individual needs? This is not rational behavior on their part. Why should they finance a learning curve when there are no immediate nor guaranteed profits? Let someone else do the research, and maybe HMOs will cover treatments when they are proven cost-effective. HMOs who do this are called "free riders."

INFORMED CONSENT

Doctors are told to prescribe the cheapest options covered by health policies. Often, you are not told of expensive therapies with better outcomes or promising experimental procedures. This concept is known as gag clauses. Shouldn't you have the right to know? What if you decide to raise the money for treatment yourself? Ethically, you have a right to know your options when you are making life and death decisions.

DILUTED COVERAGE

Soon, all plans will begin to look alike. Since cost is the priority, quality is not a driving factor. HMO premiums must be lower than their competitors'. Over time, this encourages less services to be covered. Usually, quality of life services are dropped first. An example is a knee arthroscopy to restore your ability to play golf or tennis. But your ability to play golf is not important to your HMO. It is only a matter of time before the best plans will be forced to trim extra benefits in order to compete.

RATIONING

HMOs have many ways to ration care under their definition of "efficient" care. HMOs can delegate most of the risks, yet are not governed or held to standards. Their primary business is to protect the assets of the company, and protect lives secondarily. Why wouldn't HMOs take advantage of these profitable situations?

THE CHALLENGE

The old system of fee-for-service rewards physicians for over-treatment. Since providers are paid for everything they do, there is an economic incentive to do more. By reversing this incentive, however, capitation rewards under-treatment. Capitated providers are paid to take care of populations. The number of services delivered is up to them. If the services are not delivered, they can pocket the premiums. Since each service adds costs, there is an economic incentive to do less. You as a patient can be harmed in either system. You can receive services you do not need or you can be denied services you truly need. In capitated health care plans, under-treatment is defined as:

- ▲ difficulty or inability to access a primary physician,
- ▲ deferred hospitalization,
- ▲ shortened length of hospital stays,
- ▲ referrals that are difficult, postponed, or omitted, and
- ▲ decline of quality in care.

MONITORS

There is an answer. Under-treatment is preventable using modern technology to monitor outcomes, compile satisfaction surveys, and use of case management principles. Practice protocols are available, even to consumers. These protocols are called "cookbook medicine." Practice protocols are the treatment or "recipe" for a given diagnosis. If you know your diagnosis, you can research your recommended treatment. To find a protocol for asthma, for example, go on-line at the public or medical library. Use keywords like "asthma" and "protocol" to find your disease management protocol. Now you know your treatment. And you know what to expect and what will be covered. Your provider's job is to diagnose and make sure you follow the average recovery. If you are having complications, you will need another diagnosis and protocol to follow. By knowing more about your disease and its management, you can monitor your own outcomes. You can hold your HMO, physician, and hospital accountable as things occur, not after it is too late.

References

CHA & CMCC (Date Unknown). *A Workbook for Understanding Capitation.* Catholic Health Association and Catholic Managed Care Consortium.

O'Reilly, B. (8-17-98). "What Really Goes On in Your Doctor's Office?" *Fortune.*

CHAPTER 8

On Whose Side Is Your Case Manager?

And How Is Care Managed?

What is a case manager? A case manager is your health care policy liaison, mediator, and disease management expert. This person is assigned to you by your HMO or hospital. This person helps you meet your health care needs wherever you are in the system: the clinic, hospital, or using home health services. You should get to know your case manager as well as you know your doctors. Once you understand how case management works, you can expect fewer complications and fewer denials of health coverage.

HISTORY

Case management developed in response to managed care. Before cost containment, patients would stay in the hospital for a week to 10 days. Imagine the bills for that, especially Medicare and Medicaid patients. Changes were needed. In the 1980s, the government established DRG guidelines for the number of days patients should stay in the hospital. Now, each diagnosis has a specified length of stay. For example, gallbladder surgery is a one-day procedure. Therefore, Medicare pays for the outpatient costs whether you stay for one day or three. Insurances followed this practice of limiting payments for inpatient stays or denying coverage. This forced hospitals to become more efficient.

With managed care, things are changing. HMOs prepay for your health care. Every month, your HMO pays your hospital network to provide your health care services. And you must use the hospital where the contract was made. A set fee per person is paid to the hospital whether you use health care or not. HMOs pay cash up front every month. Therefore, they can negotiate huge discounts for the people they represent. Hospitals and clinics must compete for those lives. Hospitals, therefore, are at the mercy of HMOs who control patients. They must accept discounted contracts, despite trying to make a profit. They want the small monthly fees, but their best interest is to keep you from getting sick. They will do everything to prevent hospitalizations so they can keep all the money. Instead, hospitals treat patients through outpatient or alternative services. If patients are admitted, hospitals assign case managers who coordinate your discharge as early as possible while finding alternative ways to meet your needs.

SEAMLESS SUPPORT

A case manager is a nurse, social worker, or specially trained person hired by a hospital or HMO. Their job is to see that you are not over- or under-using your benefits. If you are hospitalized, they make sure you are discharged on time. Whatever the average length of stay for your diagnosis is, that is when you go home. If you need further treatment, they arrange the following kinds of support you may or may not need.

- ▲ People support: such as physical therapy, respiratory therapy, and nurses who make house calls through home health agency arrangements.
- ▲ Equipment support: such as leased or rented equipment, crutches, wheelchairs, or home oxygen.
- ▲ Other support: such as will you have difficulty filling prescriptions? Your insurance may have specific guidelines for where your prescriptions are filled or using generic brands.

A case manager can help with who, when, where, how, and why.

PROTOCOLS

Case managers can help you with your disease protocols. They have access to information about diseases, diagnoses, and their outcomes.

Over time, statistics have been collected about patients' reactions to treatments for each diagnosis. Standards of care or protocols have been designed for patient care. For example, the number one cause of American adult illness is heart disease. A common procedure for coronary artery disease is Coronary Artery Bypass Graft (CABG). There are CABG protocols prescribing what you need each day if you have this procedure. Departments such as lab, x-ray, and physical therapy have requirements by day. By mapping out daily activities, costs can be predetermined. Knowing daily routines and daily costs automatically sets a length of hospital stay. This is the equivalent of assigning a price tag to each diagnosis. Once costs are known, budgeting is more accurate. Sometimes when HMOs negotiate for prepaid health care, they compare the costs of procedures among hospital networks. Contract negotiation becomes shopping around and comparing price tags. This is true, especially of carve-out packages.

Using protocols or pathways is not new. Remember DRGs, when limits were placed for government and poverty patients' diagnoses? These were based on average length of stays for

---

CARVE-OUT PACKAGES

Some hospitals do not offer every service or specialty. One service not offered by every hospital is organ transplant.

Your HMO wants the best deal for the most services, so it contracts with the cheapest hospital. If a carve-out is needed, your HMO will purchase a package from a center who does transplants. A center that does more transplants can offer cheaper and better carve-out packages.

diseases and average services consumed. This prevented runaway spending of government funds. Eventually, other health care insurers cashed in on this idea. This was when insurers began auditing medical bills for denying payments. They would not cover anything outside an average treatment protocol without a reasonable explanation.

This is how DRGs begat protocols. And the uses for protocols have grown. Once your doctor pronounces a diagnosis, it is entered into your electronic chart for the entire network to see. With established protocols, your network can predict you and your provider's every move. Everyone knows what will happen next. Everyone, it seems, but patients.

OUTCOMES MANDATED BY THE NCQA

If protocols are used for efficient care, why not use them to measure effectiveness? This is more difficult to visualize. For one thing, how is effective care defined? One way is to look at how patients respond to care. These responses are known as outcomes. Measuring and monitoring outcomes is one way to tell if quality care is being delivered. For example, if many patients are showing adverse outcomes to a protocol over time, then something is wrong. Something may be missing from the protocol algorithm. Currently, all facilities must measure and report outcomes to the NCQA. Then, the NCQA interprets these outcomes.

The National Commission for Quality Assurance (NCQA) identifies and accredits institutions who have the best outcomes. This stamp of approval indicates higher standards in health care. An outcome example might be monitoring birth weights of newborns. If an institution reports low birth weights consistently, then their network might need better prenatal care up-front. Or perhaps their clinics need to retool their smoking cessation classes in their prenatal programs. Critical adjustments are made for institutions with geographical, social, cultural, and severity of illness considerations.

This shatters the myth that cost and quality are impossible to separate. Case managers are instrumental in knowing the protocols, then collecting and measuring outcomes. Each case manager is responsible for a certain floor, department, or set of patients. An average case load is 20–25 patients. When you are admitted to the hospital, your case manager begins discharge planning on day one for any anticipated services you require. The manager contacts your health care plan and obtains coverage specifics. Immediately, you and your family members are made aware of alternatives and choices to be made. Daily visits are made by your case manager and variations from the protocols are captured, whether positive or negative. The goal is to provide faster, efficient yet effective and quality care.

HOW TO TAKE MORE RESPONSIBILITY IN YOUR CARE

When you visit the clinic or hospital, ask your case manager for your disease protocol or pathway. You will be given a simplified copy outlining your daily expectations and your future goals. You should become actively accountable for your progress. For example, hospitalized patients could get themselves up at 8 A.M., perform their exercises, and check off daily goals. Competition to beat deadlines amongst roommates with similar surgeries has even been seen.

HOLDING TREATMENT CENTERS ACCOUNTABLE

In addition to pathways or protocols, your network will have an information system that does many complex things.

- ▲ Code your transition through the protocol
- ▲ Complex statistical processing
- ▲ Electronic submission of outcomes to the NCQA

Your chance to communicate your opinion of protocols or outcomes comes when you are given a patient satisfaction survey. Try to complete this honestly and return it as soon as possible. This is your report of your progress to your network and, in turn, the NCQA. If you forget or neglect it, the network must rely on your case manager's documentation, or the opinion of some other stranger in your case.

DISADVANTAGES OF CASE MANAGERS

Unfortunately, there are things you need to know about case managers. Who does your case manager work for: you, the HMO, or hospital? In other words, whose interests are being protected? Are case managers helping to get you out so that the hospital is making money at your expense? Are you getting all your benefits? Are you getting quality services if you are discharged early? Case managers are expected to help you, yet they are being paid to cut costs and save money. Here are some suggestions to prevent you from getting hurt, physically and financially.

▲ The best case manager to have is one with a license. A nurse has a medical background and is better able to predict your needs. Also, a nurse will know how to avoid complications. And because of licensure, (s)he can be held legally accountable if abuse or neglect occurs.

▲ Use more than one case manager. If your insurance and hospital offer case management, use both of them. They are doing their jobs for the insurance and the hospital, and you are entitled to their services. However, they are looking after the interests of someone else; you should be looking after yours. Listen to what they propose and list options from both. Compare, contrast, make verifying phone calls, and think about each set of options. Then use the best alternatives for your situation.

▲ Be open minded to the case manager. This person has the information and power to help you. Be aware, honest, and verbalize your needs. Communication is as important with your case manager as it is with your surgeon. If you have a complex medical past, say so. This person can give guidance to prevent complications, but only if s(he) knows your history.

ADVANTAGES OF CASE MANAGERS

Two advantages to case managers are that they are on top of things, and they shoulder much of the responsibility. Take advantage of this, but stay informed. If you are uncomfortable about a decision, try to negotiate for an additional diagnosis. Pressure to meet hospital discharge requirements sometimes results in premature discharges. These are unscheduled readmissions that occur within one month of an earlier discharge. Premature discharges must be reported and analyzed. If complications could have been prevented, or another diagnosis is missed, responsibility is assigned and penalties assessed on the physician who is responsible.

CONCEPTUAL FLAWS

Some insurance plans will pay for readmission if there is no connection with early discharge. This has lead to creative diagnosing and fraudulent billing due to flaws in DRGs and pathway designs. Naively, patients are assumed to have only one problem at a time requiring treatments within the context of that problem. However, humans have many organs that attempt to compensate. Therefore, many things can go wrong at one time. Complex humans do not always categorize into simple, black and white DRGs. Several diagnoses or multiple problems may occur simultaneously. In attempting to push such a person through a tightly designed protocol, complications arise that require treatments beyond the established guidelines. The challenge to you and your doctor is to accurately diagnose and combine protocols if necessary. This is where things get complex. But don't worry, certain procedures can be done at home. Intravenous (IV) medications can be arranged on an outpatient basis or through a home health nurse.

The ethics of skirting DRG and pathway issues are debated in the literature today. With prepaid health care, no one has answers, only opinions. Higher premiums are the answer for some, but are not favorable to everyone involved.

Protocols and case managers include many challenges. An obvious issue is someone looking over the shoulders of physicians. To physicians it is frustrating, but this can be an advantage to patients. Published pathway information is available on-line, and in most medical book stores. Finding the information may be easier than following and understanding how the concept and system is intended to work. Don't hesitate to write your questions on your protocol and telephone for answers.

There is one caveat to using protocols. Guidelines are not and should not become absolutes. It is in the best interest of science to continually question practice standards. This, too, will involve costs.

CONCLUSION

In summary, HMOs set premiums that are paid to hospitals and clinics. Then, under this umbrella, protocols and pathways set costs of diagnoses and establish disease management. Once costs are established, expenses are known up-front. Easier planning makes the process more efficient. Once your diagnosis is known, the whole process is set in motion. The next step is measuring the outcomes with regional and national comparison.

Cooperative efforts in collecting and sharing outcomes is enabling national standards that dictate medical practices. This prevents premature discharges and encourages the delivery of quality health care. Currently, protocols are a universally accepted approach to measure outcomes. In addition, protocols define a *minimum* of quality care and set limits to where corners can no longer be cut.

References

Austin, C. (1988). "History and Politics of Case Management." *Generations, 12,* (5), 7–10.

Kane, R. (1988). "Case Management: Ethical Pitfalls on the Road to High Quality Managed Care." *Quality Review Bulletin, 14,* (5), 161–166.

CHAPTER 9

On Whose Side Is the Federal Government?

How Is Rationing Used?

FEDERAL GOALS

There are two federal goals in designing health care: efficiency and equity. Equity refers to the fairness used when health care is distributed among populations. Since equity is difficult to define and measure, Congress has focused on efficiency. We all agree that HMOs have proven to be efficient, but how are patients treated fairly or equally? Currently, HMOs have too much power and too much information. But with regulation, perhaps HMOs could be tolerated.

ASYMMETRIC INFORMATION

Knowledge creates power. Some of last generation's providers abused their knowledge by inducing demand: ordering unnecessary tests and defrauding insurances and the government. Unfortunately, today's providers shoulder this blame. Congress has attempted to level the playing field by transferring power to the more efficient HMOs.

Now HMOs have the power of information. Previously, HMOs had unethical gag clauses that prevented patients from learning about expensive therapies. We are seeing some gag clauses being reversed. Still, HMOs know and deny coverage for expensive disease management, such as in HIV and cancer. When one side has more information than another, they have unfair advantages. They can rewrite health policies to be more profitable. Meanwhile, the general public knows less about medical reimbursement strategies. This is why health care needs to be regulated. Patients must have symmetrical information in order to make life and death decisions.

Asymmetric information is evidence why health care can never be a normally functioning market. To protect the public, the government must police health care entities in some form.

SUPPLY AND DEMAND

The inconsistency between supply and demand explains some of the problem. Health care as a commodity is scarce. And our current method of health care coverage inflates demand. People perceive health care as free. This encourages creates greater use of it than if patients paid for it themselves. If supply is limited and demand is high, costs increase. And rationing becomes necessary.

RATIONING

The role of the government is to redistribute wealth. Taxes generate money to support social programs for the non-wealthy. When taxes are unpopular and social programs too costly, rationing becomes an alternative. Here are some popular ways to ration health care (Klein, Day, & Redmayne, 1996). Some are used in tandem.

- ▲ *Rationing by denial.* The is the most brutal and visible form of rationing. Patients are turned away because they are not suitable, or their needs are not urgent enough. The beauty of this method is that eligibility can be redefined regularly to match supply and demand. Policies can be written to exclude specific types of patients, diseases, and interventions that are subject to change without notice.
- ▲ *Rationing by selection.* This is the opposite of denial, but has the same effect. Patients are selected who use less benefits and yield higher profits. HMOs like to select healthy patients such as employees.

- *Rationing by deflection.* Instead of outright denial, patients are steered toward other programs or services. This is also known as dumping the problem in the lap of someone else. By forcing referrals, gatekeeping, and transferring risk to providers, HMOs can deflect health care services.

- *Rationing by deterrence.* This is making the process more difficult by constructing barriers. Examples are prior authorization, establishing co-payments, and creating difficulty in accessing the system. System agents are not helpful, dismissive, cold, and have no information available. If forms are available, they are incomprehensible. Lines are long and in dismal surroundings.

- *Rationing by delay.* Once access to the system has been achieved, demand can be discouraged with other options. Appointments are made for months later. There are waiting lists for surgery. Your endurance may be tested by delays, requests for more information or visits, or endless proof of documentation.

- *Rationing by dilution.* The scale and depth of services are reduced. As with socialized medicine, no one is excluded but everyone gets less. Doctors see twice as many patients in half the time. If quantity cannot be reduced, quality is diminished.

- *Rationing by termination.* The case manager declares your case closed. You are discharged from the hospital prematurely. Your employer or health care insurance drops your coverage completely.

- *Rationing by protocols or guidelines.* When protocols are established for each diagnosis, they can be prioritized and studied for cost-effectiveness. More expensive therapies will not be offered.

▲ *Rationing by muddling through.* This covers other illogical or inconsistent methods used. One of these methods is the limited right to sue hospitals and doctors or appeal. Even outside the managed care world, Congress has proposals in review to limit health care spending by placing caps on litigation awards. This is illogical because it encourages inferior care.

RATIONING THAT INCREASES SUPPLY

Rationing has advantages and disadvantages. Here is a positive situation created by rationing by dilution. On August 5, 1997, Clinton signed a reconciliation spending bill with the provision to pay nurse practitioners to treat Medicare patients. The government appears to be rationing health care to Medicare patients. But is health care diluted when advanced practice nurses provide primary health care?

Nurse practitioners can prescribe medications. Using the same protocols as physicians, these nurses order the same tests, diagnose the same diseases, prescribe the same medications, and teach the same concepts as physicians. And nurses will work for less money than physicians. This sets a precedent. HMOs, Medicaid, hospitals, and clinics are using nurses to deliver primary care, also. Nurses represent an economically efficient way to deliver scarce health care resources. And by removing legislative barriers, the government creates access to primary care for more Medicare and, potentially, other patients. This legislation makes it economically attractive for nurses to practice in rural areas where health care had not been available *previously*. Although this appears to be rationing by dilution, health care is extended and access broadened. Health care supply is increased.

Will people benefit or be hurt by this legislation? It appears that physicians will suffer from this new rule. Nurses are given a competitive means to enter the primary health care market. Why didn't the American Medical Association (AMA) lobby to prevent passage of this legislation?

- ▲ One assumption is that Medicare patients are not profitable or desirable to physicians. This is no longer true. All health care insurers now limit health care reimbursement. Congress and the president have taken legislative action to fill primary physicians slots with nurses. Medicare represents a guaranteed source of income. Nurse practitioners now compete with physicians for employment.

- ▲ Another assumption is that the AMA did lobby, but was unsuccessful. Have both physicians and the AMA lost bargaining power with the government? Have advanced practice nurses gained this power? Or is the government trying new methods to cut health care costs while increasing access? Although the intent of this law is unknown, the effects are not. Competition is invoked. The self-interests of physicians are affected. Physicians must serve customers *better* or lose Medicare reimbursements to nurses. Medicare patients may now enjoy a buyer's market.

- ▲ Patients still retain the right to choose from whom to receive primary care, a nurse provider or physician. With this new law, Medicare patients have been given more choices, especially in underserved areas. Nurse provider clinics will appear in untapped Medicare markets. Patients are not forced to see nurses. Patients still remain the judges of whom they choose as primary health care providers. This encourages honest and sincere competition for patients.

ADVANTAGES OF NURSES AS PRIMARY CARE PROVIDERS

▲ Historically, these nurses have smaller practices. Therefore, clinic congestion may be avoided by seeing nurse providers. Symptoms may be treated faster. And again, using the same protocols, nurses order the same tests, diagnose the same diseases, prescribe the same medications, and teach the same as physicians. More time for patients allows for better quality of care services.

▲ A large number of nurse practitioners are female. Women with gynecologic or obstetric conditions (Medicare coverage or otherwise) will have a greater selection of female providers. To some, this benefit may be perceived as better quality.

▲ Sometimes, patients are less intimidated by nurses and will ask more questions. Knowing more about disease will lead to better compliance. Informed and compliant patients consume less services. To some degree, less medical resources will be consumed.

DISADVANTAGES OF NURSES AS PRIMARY CARE PROVIDERS

▲ A nurse is limited in his or her scope of practice. This means complicated cases must be referred. Social costs accumulate. This means lost diagnosis time, additional waiting room time, frustration in not knowing diagnoses, and other costs that incur while waiting to see a physician. However, how different is this situation from present gatekeeping methods? Aren't there similar delays when patients with complications are referred to specialists?

▲ Elderly patients have more chronic illnesses. Patients with chronic illnesses consume large amounts of health care. Is the government using nurses to ration complicated elderly care? When nurses encounter chronic care complications, there will be rationing by deflections, delays, and deterrents. Again, how different is this situation from present gatekeeping methods? Similar deflections, delays, and deterrents occur when physicians refer patients with complications to specialists. Using this logic, how different are the goods and services of a nurse provider from those of a physician?

Access has increased, not decreased. And over time, the government will save more money rather then spend it. I argue that money is saved, not through rationing but through prevention. More money is allocated for access to primary care. If more money is spent up-front, then less is spent later in acute and expensive complications. Using nurses to emphasize primary care may actually slow the rate of Medicare spending. This benefits all who pay taxes.

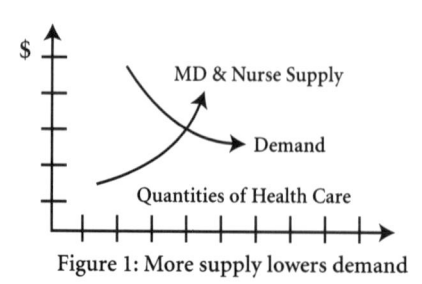

Figure 1: More supply lowers demand

This law increases the supply of health care by creating more access to primary heath care providers. Over time, the supply curve will shift up and to the right (see Figure 1). Economic theory says that as supply increases, demand relaxes. Health care prices should drop. Will too many suppliers create less demand?

No, patients want more health care if someone else pays for it. This is "moral hazard" coined by economists (Phelps, 1997).

When demand is inflated, the demand curve shifts up and to the right, see Figure 2. An inflated demand means supply needs to be higher. If the government reacts to an inflated demand by increasing the supply of providers, does the government encourage moral hazard?

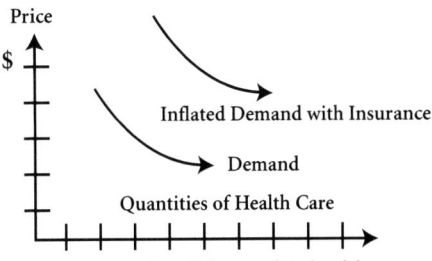

Figure 2: Inflated demand in health care

No, utilization reflects supply, not demand. When there are no providers, there are no patients. Increasing or creating additional supply will create its own demand. High rates of utilization will result. This benefits Medicare patients but *appears* to cost the taxpayers money. However, this reflects costs of primary preventative care. This cost-effective care will prevent chronic illnesses or emergency care to be incurred later.

The elderly population is increasing. Meanwhile, the taxpaying population will decrease as baby boomers retire (Wattenberg, 1997). This legislation increases supply to meet a growing future demand. In addition to increasing supply, nurse providers represent a less expensive way to provide health care. Nurses are paid less than physicians.

INCREASING COMPETITION IN HEALTH CARE

One common economic principle is that competitive markets lead to economic efficiency.

- ▲ Competition for Medicare patients forces economic efficiency. This government stamp of approval entices Medicare, HMOs, and networks to use advanced practice nurses. Nurses offer primary care at a lower price. Physicians must become more efficient or lose Medicare reimbursements to nurses.

▲ There are fewer hazards when using nurse providers. Nurses have no financial incentives to limit services, gatekeep, or induce demand. Therefore, nurses have no reason to over-treat or under-treat. Medicare patients are guaranteed a minimum standard of care. Nurses use medical resources efficiently, the government reaps in cost-benefits, and the public pays less in taxes.

▲ Again, this law emphasizes the importance of prevention. If current methods of disease prevention were applied, $1.3 billion and 80,000 deaths could be prevented every year (Vickery, 1995). Although these statistics represent national estimates, a portion relates to Medicare. In addition to saving money and lives, other positives are generated. These intangible measures are disease-free years, perception of well-being, level of activity, and quality of life.

MYTHS AND REBUTTALS TO DILUTING CARE

▲ Advanced nursing practices are a threat to physician practices. Health care is a monopolistic competition. Physicians have a monopoly to some degree, although there are competitive specialties among providers. Physicians can offer more services than these nurses: complicated treatments, minor and major surgeries, and inpatient admissions. However, physicians may do more of these services if nurses assume primary care roles. Nurses can free physicians to perform more financially rewarding procedures. This may be a disadvantage to some physicians, but could be advantageous to others. Physicians could use nurses as symbiotic partners. These two disciplines can define their roles, complement each other's schedules, and see more patients, efficiently.

▲ Decreased medical school and increased nursing school applications leads to eventual saturation of nurse providers. Is this is a potential problem for nursing schools and the nursing industry? No, nursing schools will have more choice in selecting the best and brightest students. In the long run, nursing standards will be raised and society benefits.

▲ Increased health care expenditures will result. As described, an increased supply of providers could lead to increased utilization, encouraging moral hazard. Although the supply for primary care and prevention is growing, so is demand. If growing demand or increased chronic disease is managed effectively, a more positive perception of health occurs. If Medicare patients have more opportunities to obtain primary or preventative care, they remain more active and use less cost-intensive services.

Nurses represent an economically efficient way to provide primary health care to Medicare and other patients. The government creates greater access to preventative care.

In addition to encouraging prevention, this law provides financial incentives for hospitals, clinics, managed care organizations, and other third-party payers to use nurses as primary health care providers. If more access and choices are created, the rationing debate is weakened. Rural areas may now have health care, when previously they had none.

Physicians may argue that their situation has worsened. Currently, physicians have little time to see all their patients. Nurses may offer relief. A utilitarian approach is to provide the greatest amount of good for the greatest amount of people.

Physicians are the smaller group when compared to improving the Medicare society with access and choice. However, because the elderly represents the largest and fastest growing part of our population, over time, all of society benefits.

WHAT HAPPENS IF HMOS ARE FORCED TO TAKE ON HIGH-RISK PATIENTS?

"Kennedy-Kassenbaum" (KK) went into effect on August 21, 1996. This law foreshadows what could happen when the health care bill of rights is passed. Prior to KK, insurers did not have to sell policies to high-risk patients. Since then, denying coverage for preexisting conditions is outlawed. In addition to covering chronically ill patients, insurance companies must now insure individuals whose coverage has been terminated, and small employer groups. Smaller groups offer less power to negotiate for discounts, unknown risks, and more paperwork for no profit. And individuals with terminated coverage means bigger payouts.

This law means insurance companies have two options: raise rates or find creative ways to avoid insuring high-risk groups. Since raising rates alienates customers, the latter choice has been carried to an extreme. It seems health insurance agents who sell high-risk policies are denied their commissions.

But why shouldn't high-risk people pay more for premiums if they use more health care? Because people are sensitive to the price of health care insurance. When costs are too high, people will go without. But then when catastrophes occur, the state pays for disability care under Medicaid. But wasn't the reason for this law to relieve the burden on the state? Most likely, Congress had the states in mind with this legislation (and the desire to keep high-risk voters alive). State motivations are to avoid paying for high-risk health care. State budgets are tight and risk is undesired. But, if people start to avoid insurance, we revisit the scenario of open state checkbooks for catastrophic events.

The ill cannot afford to pay the high premiums necessary to support a profitable insurance industry. Prices must be kept low to attract customers. And no insurance company can be expected to give policies gratis. They are there to make money. If there are no profits, no one will stay in the insurance business. Guess what, the private health insurance industry is not viable for the long term. Forcing insurers to take expensive cases leads private insurers to become an endangered species. This is what sparked the formation of HMOs.

The moral of the story in this case is foreboding. One lesson is that health care premiums can never go too high. Employers will not provide it as your benefit if it eats into their profits or puts them out of business. And not everyone will buy expensive health care policies. People will go without health care insurance if it becomes unaffordable.

This could happen when HMOs are forced to take on higher risk patients.

References

Foster, R. (1987). "Welfare Economics and Market Failure." Unpublished Information.

Helmlinger, C. (September/October, 1997). "American Nurses Association Hails Passage of Medicare Reimbursement." *The American Nurse.*

Klein, R., Day, P., & Redmayne, S. (1996). *Managing Scarcity: Priority Setting in the National Health Service.* Philadelphia, PA: Open University Press.

Phelps, C. (1997). *Health Economics (2nd Ed.).* New York, NY: Addison-Wesley Educational Publishers, Inc.

Vickery, D. & Lynch, W. (1995). "Demand Management: Enabling Patients to Use Medical Care Appropriately." *JOEM, 37,* (5), 1–7.

Wattenberg, B. (11-23-97). "The Population Explosion Is Over." NY: *The New York Times Magazine.*

CHAPTER 10

Where Do You Draw the Line?

What About Standards or Quality Care?

Some of you have health care horror stories. Many have tried to alert government or health care officials. Unfortunately, few are moved by subjective accounts of managed care victims. What moves officials is hard facts. Data. Statistics are what moved officials to adopt managed care initially. And slow changes in the statistics have kept managed care in business.

DRAWING BOUNDARIES IN EFFICIENCY AND EQUITY

Your employer is motivated to buy cheap health care for you. Meanwhile, the government has a limited amount of money budgeted for socialized health care. From this, government patients must get their fair share. The ideal system includes two things: efficiency and equity. It is easy to mandate efficiency. HMOs are proof that low-cost health care can be delivered to many people. But there is no way to mandate fairness or equity. The definition of fairness is too subjective and the government knows this. This is the reason HMOs continue to rule. HMOs are efficient.

However, an effort toward standards in health care is in progress. Establishing and reinforcing standards is slow and expensive. It will be difficult to reallocate, rearrange, and redistribute health care monies. Most difficult will be defining and enforcing "just the right amount" of care.

SIGNS OF CRISES IN HEALTH CARE

- ▲ *17.4% of the population is uninsured, or approximately 43,000,000.*
- ▲ *18.1% of the GNP will be spent on health care in 2000, with current spending patterns.*
- ▲ *There is a geographical maldistribution of providers.*
- ▲ *Primary and preventative care services are underutilized.*
- ▲ *There is a high rate of inappropriate utilization of health services.*
- ▲ *There are gaps in our present delivery system that prevent continuity of care.*
  - *—Patient care costs are 16% while administrative costs are 84%.*
  - *—In a four-day inpatient hospitalization, a patient interacts with 60 different employees.*
  - *—Providers and patients have differing opinions. For example, patients do not want to get lost in the system. Providers want to control patient care again. Both focuses are similar, yet how are the two working together?*

(The Robert Wood Johnson Foundation)

DRAWING BOUNDARIES IN OUTCOME MEASURES

The National Committee for Quality Assurance (NCQA) is an independent nonprofit employer-led consortium for quality health care. The NCQA has devised a minimum set of quality standards called HEDIS.

> ## WHAT IS HEDIS?
>
> *HEDIS stands for Health Plan Employer Data and Information Set. The NCQA collects HEDIS outcomes or statistics to assess health plans yearly. These statistics cover specific and general aspects of patient care.*
>
> - ▲ *Immunization rates*
> - ▲ *Breast cancer screens*
> - ▲ *Eye exams for diabetics*
> - ▲ *Smoking cessation*
> - ▲ *Cesarean section rates*
> - ▲ *Patient satisfaction*
> - ▲ *Over 300 other outcomes*
>
> *Regions of the country are scored on how well they address these issues. Then they are compared on a national basis. Consumers can obtain report cards or on-line graphs showing the best areas of the country to get health care, defined by: access, outcomes, and patient satisfaction.*

Most information is derived from existing claims data or electronic medical records. An HMO cannot compete without reporting HEDIS outcomes to the NCQA. Theses measures are compared to best practice standards. Then, the NCQA accredits health plans. *Plans that are not accredited by the NCQA should be avoided.* The NCQA seal of approval is required by employers such as GM and Xerox (Schonfeld, 1998).

Ask your employer or union if your managed care plan is accredited by the NCQA. This might be a good place for you to begin in improving your own health care benefits.

CHALLENGES IN COLLECTING OUTCOMES

Some providers think outcomes are just a new buzzword for research. Before managed care, we used methods of inquiry to guide practices; now, we use outcomes. However, research monies are shrinking to the extent that research is becoming a luxury. If research and outcomes are truly similar, will outcomes follow this dying path?

Patient satisfaction must be included in outcomes assessment. If patients are consumers, health care delivery should be measured by whether or not the consumer receives the services that (s)he expects.

But there is another problem with outcomes. Clinicians treat patients and then measure outcomes. How might outcomes take on biases to make each clinician's results look better? How can subjective results, such as patient satisfaction, be compared globally? And how are adverse outcomes acknowledged?

HOW IS QUALITY MEASURED IN HEALTH CARE?

- *LOS (patients' Length of Stays in treatment facilities)*
- *QA (Quality Assurance programs), TQM (Total Quality Management), or benchmarking programs*
- *Report Cards*
- *Outcomes, number of lawsuits, patient deaths*
- *Employee turnover in health-related occupations*
- *Customer Satisfaction Surveys*
- *Cost-Effective Analyses*

ACKNOWLEDGING ADVERSE OUTCOMES

Capitation ignores adverse outcomes. Successful managed care based on capitation theory assumes that all its members are healthy. It assumes that every procedure or surgery will have a normal recovery period and no complications. Hospitals are responsible to cover the costs of health care with complications. If a complication occurs, the hospital eats the costs. And hospitals are on shaky ground. This does not make sense. Why are complications the fault of hospitals? Why must hospitals close, make severe cutbacks, or join networks to stay afloat?

A major flaw in managed care theory occurs by assuming that human organisms are not mortal. Body systems decline over time and eventually fail. When one body system has a problem, other systems are affected. And some patients have more than one problem. Proof is in the number of medications taken by each patient. Usually, different pills are taken to alleviate different problems. Therefore, to assume that every patient with a similar diagnosis has the same needs or even average needs is wrong. Every patient

---

HOW ACTUARIES SET YOUR PREMIUMS

Setting premiums is easier than playing poker. Based on gaming, odds, probabilities, and statistics, actuaries make a living off tracking health care usage. They figure and predict utilization and then sell this information. They are not afraid of risk because they know how often people use health care and how often complications occur. Then they pad complication rates with a safety net to cover a margin of error. All this is done with computer software.

Their expertise lies in the ability to exploit this information. Once you know probabilities of how much health care will be used, you spread the costs over the people covered.

should receive individualized care according to his or her needs. Capitation works in theory but not in practice.

Adverse outcomes occur with statistical regularity. Using a normal bell-shaped curve and healthy patients, a majority of outcomes are positive all of the time. But a minority of outcomes will be negative all of the time. Allowances must be figured for the probabilities of these negative outcomes. This is where actuaries are useful. They determine fair health care premiums based on these and other assumptions.

Some HMOs do not use actuaries to set their premiums. This means adverse outcomes may not be built into your premiums.

The United States is seeing the majority of the population growing older and developing chronic health care problems. This means outcomes will grow less positive over time. Resources for adverse outcomes must be predicted and allowances built into health care premiums. This needs to occur now, before it is too late for hospitals.

LONG-TERM EFFECTS

Capitation acts as a parasite to everyone in an integrated network. In addition to alienating patients, managed care plans cannot continue to alienate providers and hospitals. If long-term relationships are to be maintained, MCOs must protect their patients and their networks. In their current state, HMOs are not satisfying customers' nor their networks' needs. This is not the secret to long-term success.

OTHER LONG-TERM IMPLICATIONS

Managed care changes have occurred rapidly and extensively. Little is known about long-term effects on health care: quality, access, and costs. Meanwhile, policy makers, health and business professionals, purchasers, and consumers of health care must try to make thoughtful and reasonable decisions. Here are some other concerns.

▲ We know that newer rate-setting mechanisms ignore adverse outcomes. Not only are patients used as economic guinea pigs, but they cannot reward the best providers of care with repeat business. This is not common sense. Why must survival of the fittest determine how our health care is delivered?

▲ MCOs do not encourage future progress and access to new technology. Providers have tight protocols that do not look at methods that may work better. HMOs do not want to suffer through unknown success rates for new technology. But huge potential is created by a burgeoning technological age. How will scientific advancements be made if MCOs discourage innovation?

▲ If patients, providers, and hospitals are not involved in future medical technology decision-making, who is? Aren't health care personnel the ones who understand what innovations are needed? Why are cost-conscious administrators making these decisions?

▲ MCOs grow more and more efficient over time. Is increased efficiency due to failures of less efficient MCOs? Is it due to growing enrollment and achieving economies of scale? Or is it due to mergers leading to larger, more efficient *but less effective* MCOs? Is this a fire growing out of control? Too much efficiency leads to managed price, not managed care.

The weak link with financial people as HMO administrators is lack of quality of care issues. But the weak link with providers as HMO administrators is a lack of efficiency. Both issues must be an HMO's focus.

DRAWING LEGAL BOUNDARIES

Presently, malpractice punishments in dollar awards do not punish HMOs or practitioners. Payouts come from malpractice insurance. Therefore, reproaches are not felt internally. Different options are needed to encourage ethical behavior, intellectual growth, and prevent abuses.

What are we really trying to accomplish? We need to relax the costs of defensive medicine and lower panic and litigation thresholds. We must create and share learning from mistakes, rather than cover them up. Although civil wrongs should not go unpunished, a punishment for a liable provider might be to research the mistake and propose solutions for prevention. In this way, new knowledge is generated for publication, and public policy issues are promoted in a positive light.

DRAWING ETHICAL BOUNDARIES

One missing patient right is ethical treatment for patients. Currently, there is no accountability for providers who breach medical ethics. Hospitals should have visible ethics committees or an ethical consultant on staff. This should be a contingency for accrediting hospitals. Smaller networks could have a traveling ethicist. The benefits and costs could be shared. Ethicists can raise standards in the following ways:

- ▲ Offer refresher seminars of medical ethics for health care professionals
- ▲ Help patients and their families in difficult situations make life and death decisions
- ▲ Institute, maintain, and enforce ethical standards

An HMO patient's bill of rights could hold HMOs responsible for ethics. A contingency for obtaining or retaining an HMO license would be an ethicist on staff. If unethical behaviors could be prevented up-front, litigation costs, bad outcomes, and lives might be spared.

WHAT ARE MEDICAL ETHICS?

▲ *Autonomy means patients have the right to self-determination. This includes the right to information and the right to refuse treatment. A patient can do whatever is best for his or her social, economic, mental, physical, or familial situation.*

▲ *Beneficence means a provider must do good. This includes delivering just the right amount of care—no more and no less.*

▲ *Confidentiality means providers must respect privileged information.*

▲ *Fidelity means providers must keep promises.*

▲ *Good faith means acting in the right way based on all known information.*

▲ *Justice means treating people fairly.*

▲ *Non-maleficence means providers must do no harm, actively or passively. Examples are being over-aggressive, over-conservative, or ignoring a symptom or situation.*

▲ *Respect is necessary for conducting and maintaining provider-client relationships.*

▲ *Veracity means telling the truth to peers and patients.*

These are fundamental ethical mandates that apply to all practice settings. Also, they include changing clinical realities in genetics and future technology. This framework applies to behavior across all health care professions and dimensions (Scanlon & Fibison, 1995).

DRAWING BOUNDARIES IN PROTOCOLS

Protocols must be reviewed at least yearly to include innovations, or to remove outdated or substandard actions. Procedures that are standardized risk the loss of human judgment and critical thinking. Diseases are treated and not people. Predetermined care encourages complacency and discourages innovation. Providers are no longer being paid to think, but to follow an approved list. *Managed care is practicing medicine without a license, but the providers seem to be the ones sued.* Are health care professionals allowed to do what they have been trained to do?

CONCLUSION

As things stand, HMOs are allowed to milk all facets in health care dry. When the baby boomers age, most likely the HMOs will pull out. There will be few profits to make on higher risk and chronically ill patients. Only then will the retreat of HMOs capture attentions from those in power in the same seriousness as the Savings and Loan crises. I can only hope that I am wrong.

Once, a patient looked me in the eye and said, "It's health care that needs the enema, not me." This is a bit extreme. But health care could stand a change of diet. A bill of rights or competition for consumers would make HMOs easier to swallow.

References
The Robert Wood Johnson Foundation.
Scanlon, C. & Fibison, W. (1995). *Managing Genetic Information: Implications for Nursing Practice.* Washington, DC: ANA.
Schonfeld, E. (3-30-98). "Can Computers Cure Health Care?" *Fortune.*

How Is Managed Care Creating Progress?

CHAPTER 11

Why Is Health Care For-Profit?

"...to the efficient go the increasing returns"
—Richard Arrow, Economist

Just how much success do we enjoy as a leader of industrialized nations? Standard of living is one way to measure economic success. But when standards of health care are compared across nations, perspectives change; Americans consume gluttonous amounts of health care.

The United States has all the elements of success. We have resource-generous land, adequate labor, abundant capital, and ideas from entrepreneurs. Our forefathers set up a government that encourages free enterprise, rewards for education, and tax laws favoring growing businesses. However, when work ethics run deep, so do expectations. We work hard so we can play hard. Don't we deserve to enjoy our economic success? When we are capable of cutting edge health care, shouldn't we take advantage of it?

In a normal industry, consumers drive the economy. Businesses get repeat business by catering to customers' needs. *In our country, health care is a for-profit business.* Therein lies the ambiguity. HMOs are allowed to be businesses, but patients are not allowed to drive the health care economy.

IMPLICATIONS

Adam Smith's claim to fame is as the father of economics. His "invisible hand" theory says greed is good. It fuels private enterprise and results in socially beneficial outcomes. New jobs create spending, increase living standards, and generate community growth. But again, competition for consumers is a necessary ingredient. And competition for patients is a missing link with HMOs. This has caused a market failure and government intervention is necessary. Restoring a patient's right to choice creates competition among providers. And a competing remedy would be to change tax laws to favor medical savings accounts. This would create competition *between* MSAs and HMOs. In addition, MSAs force patients to self-ration their health care.

But is managed care the enemy? HMOs have begun to train consumers in how to ration their own care. On the contrary, here is a growing list of positive changes.

- ▲ Patients stay in the hospital far fewer days.
- ▲ Many surgeries previously requiring hospitalization are safely performed in day surgery.
- ▲ There is far more attention paid to preventative care.
- ▲ Many medical practices have been standardized to produce better outcomes.
- ▲ Satisfying patients has become an explicit goal.

Perhaps a few simple regulations to managed care and MSAs create the most efficiency. All can compete. And profits are the reward for efficient and effective health care plans. Gains are felt when certain health care processes are made profitable. Health care dollars will go farther.

A LESSON LEARNED FROM CANADA

There is a growing trend to replace an organ or system when it fails. Canada has one of the worst organ donation rates in the Western world. The supply is not keeping pace with demand (*The Globe and Mail*, 1998). Why is this? Canada has socialized medicine. And there are no incentives to retrieve organs.

MAKING ORGAN DONATION SELF-SUFFICIENT

In 1987, Colorado, too, had a shortage of organ donors. However, Colorado Organ Recovery Service (CORS), now renamed, employed financial incentives to increase organ donations. CORS charged for organ recovery expenses and used the money to create a larger supply. People were hired to carry out organ awareness. The evidence was an increase in organs retrieved. Prior to this nonprofit group, the transplant market was stagnant. No one wanted to recover organs because they were expected to do it for nothing.

Reward for hard work revived a restricted market. By motivating organ retrieval with fees, procurement became self-sufficient. And opportunities for transplant expanded. Before CORS, organ recovery was done through philanthropy. By not rewarding time and skills invested in organ retrieval, there was no incentive to get organs. Without this reward for effort, apathy restricted transplant potential and the health of Colorado patients. The arrival of CORS created a healthy competition and furthered public interests in many ways.

- ▲ CORS improved transplant skills. More transplants allows specialists' skills to become proficient. Increased volume and a successful reputation improved Colorado outcomes. Outside contracts were attracted. CORS protected local interests and stimulated the economy. This illustrates Adam Smith's "invisible hand" concept.

- ▲ The cost structure of the group is nonprofit, and represents a public good. CORS generates money to finance an increased organ supply. This benefits Colorado by better satisfying demand. If a public good exists to prevent exploitation, here, the public is protected from stagnation or neglect. To a degree, the ethical principle of *justice* is served because more patients with organ failure are offered the chance to be healthy.

- ▲ To most patients, the cost of transplant is irrelevant. CORS is paid to increase the organ supply by charging transplant patients more. Patients are free not to have a transplant if costs outweigh the value of life. Since many transplants are financed by a third party, this is not an issue. Even with self-payment, patients are less sensitive to cost when the alternative is death. This makes transplant demand inelastic, regardless of a higher price.

- ▲ However, patient insensitivity to costs creates a moral hazard for those who pay the bill. Medicaid's response was regulation, and prices were fixed on kidney transplants. But in 1987, costs could be shifted to other insurance groups. Now, kidney transplants are more *cost-effective* than dialysis. An increased supply of kidneys means less dialysis. The best interest of insurers and taxpayers is to finance transplants rather than dialysis.

- ▲ More work is created for hospital staff and doctors by injecting a financial incentive into organ procurement. This advantage is a side effect from increased supply. To increase donor availability is hard work, late nights, and long hours. Proper compensation motivates this work. Those involved can quantify their worth in charges and negotiate for better salaries. Hospital staff may collect overtime. Many financial incentives are created, again, by an invisible hand. Organ retrieval must be motivating in order to grow.

Ethics are maintained by government regulation. CORS remains efficient and effective. With a sensitive subject such as a shortage of organs, introducing financial incentives with regulation was the successful way to create an organ supply.

The lesson learned is that health care can be regulated and be profitable at the same time.

MAKING ORGAN DONATION PROFITABLE

Do you think twice about exchanging car parts? Are not human parts and human life more valuable than a car? Imagine preventing needless young deaths from chronic illnesses. When we are capable of cutting edge health care, shouldn't we take advantage of it?

Someday, everyone will have routine organ transplants. The exceptions will be trauma, cancers, or other unknown disease treatments. You are probably thinking, this is ridiculous. However, consider the future treatment for burned out body parts.

If most people die of heart disease, then the new standard may be to transplant new hearts for everyone at age 50. Maybe this sounds a little extreme now, but if organs were readily available, this would be the cure for chronic disease. Rather than fight diabetes, get a new pancreas, right? Tired of asthma, get a new set of lungs. Whatever organ causes you problems, just replace it.

Nobel prizewinner Gary Becker thinks the federal government should have the authority to buy and sell organs. Whenever deaths occur, families receive $10,000 in compensation per organ rather than donate free organs. Organs donations would skyrocket. In turn, the government would sell them for a profit. This would increase the supply of organs, and profits could be used to find cures for other illnesses.

ADVANTAGES

▲ Those who need organs would be transplanted immediately.
▲ There would shorter waiting lists.
▲ More organs are available to transplant before critical tissue destruction sets in. For example, the chronically ill would be transplanted prior to major complications. These people continue to work and represent premiums

paid into HMOs, rather than draw payouts because of disability. The investment for a transplant is repaid within a few years.

▲ More money would be used in health care up-front but less in complications later.

▲ Organ research would become an industry. Every organ would be studied for transplant ability. The immunosuppression industry would mushroom. No one would die from chronic illness. Life would be prolonged. Everyone could get as many hearts as they need.

▲ It could slow the progression or even cure early cancers.

▲ Better technology will emerge exponentially.

DISADVANTAGES

▲ The poor cannot afford two to three hearts and would be eliminated sooner. The rich would stay alive longer, but pay that many more years of taxes.

▲ Black market organs will materialize. People will sell one kidney.

▲ Religious or immoral implications will arise. Strict regulation will have to be imposed.

▲ Competition for organs will exist. When transplant becomes the means for prolonging life, everyone will have programs. The industry will need intense regulation.

If this will happen someday, why not do it in your lifetime?

CONCLUSION

All pay health care premiums through employment for a working lifetime. This would cover the costs of two to three transplants per life. This would create economic efficiency in solving the donor shortage. If the public were to agree to this, all will reap the advantages. Demand could be forecasted for average survival times of each organ. Those who could afford multiple transplants could stay alive indefinitely. Imagine the social benefits and opportunity savings of keeping American knowledge and experience alive longer.

For-profit health care encourages innovation while providing the means to fund progress. And if a health care bill of rights is in place now, abuses could be prevented.

References
Becker, G. (1-20-97). "How Uncle Sam Could Ease the Organ Shortage." *Business Week*, 28.
Kassier, J. (1-6-95). "Managed Care and the Morality of the Marketplace." *NEJM 333*, (1), 50–52.
Picard, A. (7-15-98). "Supply lags demand in organ transplants." *The Globe and Mail* (Montreal, Canada Newspaper).

CHAPTER 12

What Are Alternative Solutions?

"You can always count on the Americans to do the right thing—but only after they have tried everything else…"
   —Winston Churchill (McDermott, 1995)

An HMO patient's bill of rights is not the only cure for our ailing system. There are other ideas for injecting quality back into the arms of modern health care. A bill of rights may or may not change behavior. Some argue it will force unethical behaviors underground. Loopholes will be found, for example, through ERISA. Other ways may promote change without spending too much of the patient's money, as, ultimately, the patient will be the one who pays. Again, HMOs or insurance, providers, and hospitals must be allowed to make money or no one will remain in business. Then there will be no health care.

What are alternative solutions? Here is a thumbnail sketch of other ideas. Or perhaps the answer is a combination of methods.

- ▲ Removing Conflicts of Interest for Providers
- ▲ Provider-Sponsored HMOs
- ▲ Patient-Determined Rationing with Medical Savings Accounts
- ▲ Avoidance
- ▲ Universal Coverage
- ▲ Geographically Specific Solutions

REMOVING CONFLICT OF INTEREST FOR PROVIDERS

Dr. Klass, a new pediatrician, was shadowing an internist. The purpose was to learn—not how to take care of kids—but the motivations behind capitation. The novice practitioner wanted to learn the secrets providers use to maneuver in the managed care environment. (Klass, 1997) When capitation was introduced, providers learned to behave differently. This change is better understood if placed on a spectrum. Fee-for-service, at one extreme, promotes more health care spending to get more reimbursements. The other extreme, capitation, encourages withholding health care by punishing spending. What is a provider to do? Dr. Klass' mentor had her own idea. Make providers "blind" to patient's insurance information.

If we mandate that insurance information become as confidential as a diagnosis, this will remove doctors from treating the needs of HMOs rather than the patients'. Let doctors return to practicing medicine and not politics. Then, providers have no reason to over-treat or under-treat. This puts the patient back in the foreground. Providers' thinking is not clouded by financial bonuses or penalties.

If providers have no knowledge of who is paying, gag clauses are a moot point. Full disclosure of treatment will occur because only the patient knows who and how the bill is settled. Then there is no failure to refer or to over- or under-utilize key services. Currently, there is a conflict of interest by treating the needs of the third-party payer and not the needs of patients. Full choice returns to the consumer. And this, in turn, lowers health care costs. There are no financial incentives to do more tests, as with fee-for-service. And there are no penalties for doing less, as with capitation. The solution is to find and remove conflicts of interest.

There are disadvantages. Capitation has controlled health care costs better than fee-for-service. Why? It's because patients weren't getting the right amount of treatment. If patients get the right amount of health care, more health care costs more money. But it does not cost as much the runaway train medicine, fee-for-service. Gatekeeping, if practiced, remains between the patient and the insurance company. This is as it should be. If your insurance won't cover something, let them deliver the bad news directly to you. This allows you, the patient, to ask why. This allows you to blame and switch insurers, not doctors. Why force the provider to be in the middle, to say no? Permission for access, ER visits, and other sensitive issues are between patient and insurance.

Networks still exist, acting as buying cooperatives. Purchases such as drugs can be bought in bulk, and with discounts. This relieves providers of the unrealistic expectation of knowing all guidelines of all possible health plans.

Capitation 101 is not found in modern medical school curriculums. There is a reason for this. It conflicts with the medical ethics of autonomy, beneficence, good faith, justice, non-maleficence, respect, and veracity.

PROVIDER-SPONSORED HMOS

Uwe Reinhardt thinks physicians will "take back medicine." But Doctor Reinhardt is not a physician. He is a professor of Political Economy at Princeton. He favors physician competition as a solution to capitation. Physicians must be given more incentives and advantages to run their own HMOs.

Previously, provider groups were prevented from offering health plans to patients by antitrust legislation. Now, Congress has written legislation, "exemptions to monetary reserves" for physicians to dominate managed care. Provider-Sponsored Networks (PSNs) will have no monitors or constraints placed by non-physicians. PSNs could eliminate the insurance industry as middleman and absorb those profits. Because of this future threat, insurance groups are afraid. In areas not fully capitated, HMOs are not pushing for pure capitation. HMOs are afraid PSNs will form faster and be stronger. But here are some questions that arise if providers are allowed to rule.

- ▲ Would PSNs merge with insurance groups and hospitals?
- ▲ Will they be collegial such as a Mayo Clinic by inspiring trust from patients? Or will physicians march to a financial tune?
- ▲ How different will PSNs incentives be from HMOs? What is their Achilles' heel? (See sidebar for concerns.)
- ▲ How will employers begin to contract with providers when they have asymmetrical or more knowledge on their side? Could this monopoly of knowledge that providers have lead to supply-induced demand? Would this turn back the clock to fee-for-service?
- ▲ Who will look over the shoulder of providers to prevent over-treatment or under-treatment?

THE ACHILLES' HEEL OF PSNS

PSNs are at a disadvantage. Price, not quality, is a driving force. Therefore, they may not be able to compete. Physicians will want to provide more services rather than ration. This means costs and premiums will be higher in PSNs than in financially run HMOs. Employers are looking for cheap benefits for their employees. And states, who are looking for a good deal for populations, will pass over PSNs' promises of quality care.

Unless you or your union demand better benefits, PSNs will struggle.

Health care consumers are vulnerable. Patients depend on the goodwill of health care agents to provide cost-effective coverage and care. Unfortunately, this trust is a breeding ground for exploitation and corruption. There is no perfect solution. There are too many players to please. However, if an error is made in someone's favor, it should be the greatest good for the greatest number. And the majority concerned are consumers.

CONSUMER SOVEREIGNTY

The consumer rules. (S)he is the best person to decide what (s)he needs at the time. Based on families' priorities, (s)he decides how much money is spent on health care. If a college education has to be purchased, health care may become secondary. But the consumer must live with the ramifications of decisions made. The problem with consumer sovereignty is, so do others. If childhood immunizations are ignored, disease is caught and spread. Consumers' experiences with illness are often limited. Therefore, judgments are subject to error. Parents may not make the choices that will maximize their children's welfare.

This is another reason that health care is not a normal market. Previously, physicians could act as paternalistic agents to manufacture the best outcomes for their patients. With managed care, incentives attempt to pull physicians' strings to manufacture the best outcomes for the HMOs. If physicians cannot act in good faith for patients, then who will? With health care information available today, consumer sovereignty deserves a chance.

PATIENT DETERMINED RATIONING WITH MEDICAL SAVINGS ACCOUNTS (MSAS)

There is a broad consensus among health care economists of what to do. They believe "consumer sovereignty" is the value system that should underlie health care delivery.

This is called demand-side rationing. Patients take responsibility for how much and where money is spent on health care. If consumer sovereignty and demand-side rationing are in place, consumers choose health plans, providers, and hospitals. Then, Adam Smith's "invisible hand" kicks in. Adam Smith argues that capitalism, not to be confused with capitation, is socially beneficial. The interaction between greedy individuals who build the best businesses win consumers. The consumer must be courted. The invisible hand is the positive protection for the consumer that this implies. If health care resources are scarce, let businesses use quality and cost to compete for patients. When patients cannot choose their provider or where to go, the "invisible hand" in competition is tied. Health care economists say healthy markets grow when consumers retain the right to vote with their feet. Meanwhile, capitation has removed the consumer and patient from the picture.

If demand-side rationing were practiced, patients would have a credit card account with a yearly spending limit. Or individuals could have MSAs that collect interest. These accounts could roll over every year if not used. Consumers could ration their own health care. Patients are rewarded for not using too much health care. Interest on money left over is wealth redistributed to those who use health care wisely.

> ## HOW DOES CATASTROPHIC INSURANCE WORK?
>
> *There are niches within the insurance industry. One niche caters to people who are averse to the catastrophic risks in addition to regular health coverage. In addition to receiving MSAs, this plan is purchased for patients by employers and the states. It is included as the allotment for one year's worth of health care. It is less expensive than regular health care insurance because it only kicks in after a freak accident in nature.*
>
> *Consider how often a catastrophic event occurs, such as a paralyzing injury. Statistically, probabilities are low, but catastrophes do happen with regularity. Premiums are collected on all such employees or state patients. These premiums are invested to generate interest. When a catastrophe occurs, payouts are made from this pool of money. If you opt for a catastrophic policy, be sure you are comfortable with the definition of "catastrophe." In addition to comfort with this definition, ask if there is a stop-loss clause. A stop-loss clause means after a certain dollar payout, the catastrophic policy stops. Negotiate for a dollar amount that is comfortable, also.*

How do MSAs work? MSA deposits replace previous health care insurance premiums. This account is used to pay for health care. If there are not enough funds for a catastrophe, an additional policy kicks in.

If money remains at the end of the year, it is the employee's to keep or roll over for the next year. There are motivating implications. MSAs create incentives that affect the behavior of their owners. These incentives affect how health care will be delivered.

MSAS AT A GLANCE

Advantages	Disadvantages
1. Provides an incentive to shop around for cheapest health care available.	1. Prevention and quality issues are ignored. Less incentive for second opinions.
2. Extra money belongs to the employee.	2. This is taxable income.
3. Gives more control to the patient. Individuals are empowered.	3. Uninformed patients may choose to neglect themselves or family members.
4. Low health care users are rewarded.	4. Moderate users are penalized.
5. Eliminates insurance middleman. Eliminates co-pays.	5. Providers can raise costs without a monitoring body. Large potential for exploitation exists.
6. Patients reward best providers with their repeat business.	6. Employers would be responsible for educating employees about prevention. Why should they?

MSA COMPLICATIONS

Are health care economists right? Is market-driven health care the answer based on consumerism, technology, and entrepreneuring? Already, we have discussed how health care is not just another business. It requires more regulation than fast food chains, auto, or retail sales. There must be safety nets to protect those who fall through the cracks and prevent the spread of disease. But things get even more complicated.

MSAs are popular in the Midwest. However, MSAs are new enough that motivations and behaviors are not fully known. Good and bad outcomes on families' behaviors or choices must be studied. Employees may choose not to use any health care, and pocket the money. For example, prescriptions may not be refilled so as to support smoking habits. Those with MSAs could ignore prevention programs, and use the difference to go on vacation. This puts consumers in a position to budget opportunity costs.

OPPORTUNITY COSTS

When only one opportunity can be chosen, it costs you the benefits of the lost opportunity. Lost benefits are called opportunity costs.

The same situation occurs when you are forced to choose amongst therapies. If HMOs choose therapies for you, you suffer opportunity costs. When rationing health care, opportunity costs must be considered in cost-effective formulas to prioritize treatments. (You will see the difficulties of this in Chapter 14.)

Persons who choose vacations over health care will end up with more acute and expensive illnesses later. Serious illnesses are this person's only motivation to spend money on health care. Preventative care and second opinions, previously standard items, become luxury items. Minors or the elderly who depend on others for health care decisions could be neglected. Children, elderly, and the uninformed, whose priorities are not health-related, will suffer. This creates costs for society, or what health care economists call externalities.

EXTERNALITIES

An externality is when the actions of one party affect another, but cannot be measured in dollars. Externalities can be positive or negative. An example of a negative externality is air pollution. A factory that pollutes a neighborhood could be creating lung cancer victims. When negative externalities affect society, they create social costs. When rationing health care, social costs must be considered in cost-effective formulas to prioritize treatments. (Again, you will see the difficulties of this in Chapter 14.)

Perhaps MSA money could finance a new roof. A new roof that replaces an inhalable fungus growing in the old rotten roof. The consumer decides which is the more important priority. MSAs will create lost benefits and costs to society. But HMOs do now. With MSAs, the *consumer* chooses which costs will be suffered, not the HMO.

At this time, there is no incentive to use MSAs. MSAs are taxed as income, currently, and employer-provided health care benefits are not. In addition, health care decisions are not black and white. And, consumers may not make rational nor well-informed health care decisions. Dealing with emotional issues can lead to illogical decisions. A terminal illness could lead to unrealistic hope and unrealistic spending. Sometimes the paternalistic physician model is safer when irrational behavior occurs.

With MSAs, the healthy, with few health risks, can make money on MSAs. This leaves HMOs to fight over high-risk patients. But currently, no HMOs want high-risk patients. They are too expensive for which to coordinate care. High-risk patients consume profits. There could be no other patients left for HMOs. This would lead to the demise of the HMO industry. Pools of healthy people are needed to set off the expenses of the high-risk patients. Is this why tax advantages are not passed by the government, to protect the HMO industry?

With MSAs, the government will be left to support the high-risk ill. Taxes will increase. If the government sets up MSA accounts for the poor or high risk, it is likely that no health care is used, and money is spent elsewhere. Consider the likelihood of MSA money to support drug or alcohol habits.

Currently, insurance lobbyists balance provider lobbyists. Insurance or HMOs are middlemen that look over provider's prescribing and ordering habits to prevent runaway spending. HMOs are beneficial for this reason. Insurance offsets the monopoly power of doctors. If the middle person is removed, we return to a fee-for-service arrangement. With consumer sovereignty, will providers prescribe whatever is financially best for providers? Or will competition for patients keep them fair and honest? This is a difficult mistake to make twice.

QUALITY CARE RETURNS WITH MSAS

MSAs work well if consumers are informed. The on-line population has more health care information than they can use. With the information age creating educated patients, then health care should exist between providers and patients, without middle persons. Most people can pay the bulk of their medical expenses out of pocket, leaving insurers to cover only very costly procedures. Competition for patients will engineer quality, convenience, effectiveness, and economic efficiency. In theory, competitive equilibrium will be achieved.

MORAL HAZARD RELAXES WITH MSAS

The moral hazard of health care is relieved. There is no temptation to use more health care than necessary. If we assume responsibility for our own care, more prudent decisions will be made. Demand will relax when patients assume costs. Less health care will be used. Decisions will be based on consumer sovereignty and ability to pay. This case solves the rationing problem. Cost-benefit decisions are made by health care users. There is no welfare loss because the consumer chooses when and where costs and benefits are equal. Rationing decisions are made by patients, not third parties. Consumers can blame no one but themselves.

CHOICE IS PRESERVED WITH MSAS

Patients retain choice of providers. If providers charge too much, consumers will go elsewhere. MSAs encourage people to shop around. And shopping around is what HMOs are making big bucks to do now. Quality improves if providers must compete for patients by quality and by cost. In addition, MSAs are a way to promote alternative therapies. You may see chiropractors, osteopaths, acupuncturists, nurse practitioners, or the most expensive specialist. You are not limited to one gatekeeper. Because, *you* are the gatekeeper.

Health care cannot promise cure. Patients must be allowed to find quality, cost-effective ways to relieve suffering. When human nature brings aging and death, patients must have choice in methods of relief. With fingertip education available through computer technology, Americans can individualize their own care. With you in charge of medical spending, perhaps the Rolls Royce treatment isn't desired.

- ▲ Heart patients may not want expensive bypass surgery when a cheaper cardiac catheterization (cath) can open vessels without surgery? With a cardiac cath, you go home the next day.
- ▲ Is an expensive new heart valve necessary when a balloon procedure can fix it in one day? After ballooning a valve, you need not take anticoagulants for the rest of your life.

These are a few examples how an entire MSA is not depleted. Money would be left to cover other family needs.

CONCLUSIONS DRAWN FROM MSAS

Health care is different and more complex than other industries—one where regulations cause incentive-based behavior. Currently, HMOs have introduced some efficiency, thereby slowing the rising costs of health care. However, MSAs, with tax incentives, would favor economic efficiency, but they would be consumer-driven. If tax incentives are granted, it favors provider-sponsored networks. They will have a competitive advantage. Rather than the HMOs' low prices driving competition, *quality* could return for patients.

Adam Smith would be surprised at the ironies in America. The United States prides itself on a capitalistic system. Yet, current HMO contracts and health care issues are decided without consumer involvement. The goal of health care economics is efficiency and effectiveness. Isn't the consumer the best judge of how much technology, science, or medicine (s)he is willing to buy? If efficiency and effectiveness are our goals, then the government's obligation is to establish competitive markets in health care. Give patients the power to reward the most efficient providers of care. MSAs with tax incentives seem the best consumer tool available to drive the health care market, especially for the healthy. Just as there is no single best therapy, there is no single best health care system. Even MSAs have risks and disadvantages.

AVOIDANCE

Some Americans are choosing to deal with the health care problem by avoidance. They just don't opt for health care benefits. Employers will pay better if you don't demand health care benefits. Then, in an effort to save money, these folks don't acquire coverage until too late. No prevention or early detection leads to more acute illnesses in the long run. This leads to costly emergency care for unpredictable illness later.

There are 43 million people in this position. With current distaste for managed care, this number is growing. Denial is only a short-term solution. But, don't be fooled. This is a viable option for a growing number of people. Without addressing or meeting the needs of this growing group, ignorance costs Americans more later.

But both HMOs and MSAs can mimic this problem as well. With MSAs, patients can milk their MSAs and ignore the health of their families. This precedent was set by HMOs who milk profits while ignoring the health of their patients.

GEOGRAPHICALLY SPECIFIC SOLUTIONS

Canada gives every citizen the right to health care supported through taxes. Of every Canadian dollar spent in health care, $0.98 goes to the health care providers, displaying an economically sound vehicle of care delivery (Fulton, 1994). But it is unpopular because of:

▲ high taxes,
▲ lack of quality,
▲ waiting times of 11 weeks for an appointment to see a specialist, and
▲ limited access to experimental or cutting-edge medical technology.

Other immeasurable issues are added physical pain, and time off work. This sounds similar to HMOs because both use the same rationing techniques. But in Canada consumers pay taxes rather than have their premiums paid to HMOs. If you think socialized medicine is the answer, you are living something very similar to it.

Furthermore, it is illegal to spend private funds on health care under the Canada Health Act. This is counter-intuitive because private spending saves the government money. One Montreal newspaper asks for MSAs to be allowed (*The Globe and Mail*, 1998).

Hawaii practices the path of least resistance, the employer-mandated method. This is fondly called "play or pay" by employers. Although in some states, employers who self-insure are protected by ERISA from strict state health care regulations. Working Hawaiians may retain insurance for up to six months when changing jobs, or during the unemployment process (Skolnick, 1996). With employer mandates, however, a financial burden is borne by small businesses. This has lead small business to adopt policies of retarded hiring, lay-offs, or bankruptcy, despite promises of government assistance (McIllrath, 1994).

However, in a lecture delivered by an analyst at the University of Pennsylvania's Center for Bioethics, it was argued that quality has eroded within the Canadian single-payer health care system as the result of funding cuts. The analyst stated that Canada's national government is "starving" its health care system by reducing its contribution to the provinces' systems from 50 to 25 percent, and the system covers less than 70 percent of Canada's national health costs. (Deloitte & Touche, 1998)

Minnesota is making progress, although it enjoys the second lowest percentage of uninsured in the U.S. (Greenfield, 1996). Two of many current debates in this health-pioneering state are as follows. Replace profit-centered health care with not-for-profit health centers. This stand shows a fresh and new respect toward humans. Human life is no longer viewed as a commodity of risk by which to earn unreasonably high returns. Investors with superior expectations will be directed to look elsewhere for profits. Secondly, a microcosm in its infancy, "MinnesotaCare" is a program for statewide universal coverage. Again, this is heroic because Minnesota has fewer uninsured or unemployed persons.

California physicians have maximized a statewide network of partnerships against the managed care tidal wave, with far-reaching effects and monumental ramifications. Their referrals and affiliations go to those without managed, financial, or unethical ties. They ask, are we here to exploit people or care for people? (NPR, 1997). Some PSNs are declaring bankruptcy, finding that their higher rates for quality care cannot compete when they cannot offer low rates as HMOs.

The individual-mandate method requires personal responsibility for obtaining and funding familial or coverage for oneself. This is similar to auto insurance laws where if you drive, you must have auto insurance. Fines or penalties would be levied on those who chose not to participate. Consumers could participate by various methods. Examples are MSAs, payroll deductions, and federal subsidies for those with low incomes (Tenery, 1994).

State waivers allow a state to cater to its specific needs. Minnesota can afford its program because most of the state works to fund it. Imagine this in California or New York. Hawaii is small enough that it can experiment with employers. Meanwhile, the country can watch and learn from states with the best innovations.

UNIVERSAL COVERAGE SAVES ACADEMIA

To adopt universal coverage would be to adopt the Canadian system and all its flaws. We know that managed care ignores progress in medicine. But some argue that socialized medicine is the only method that prevents the extinction of academic medicine. It preserves the missions of academic research, teaching, and charity care. And it prevents University Hospitals from competing with HMOs.

Having HMOs in power favors for-profit institutions. These institutions can provide cheaper and less complex services for profit. They do not have the added costs of research and teaching. For-profit networks use subtle methods of patient-dumping. Academic medicine cannot.

Meanwhile, federal support of academic institutions is dwindling because Congress is trying to balance the budget. Academic institutions cannot cost-shift because private insurers are not naive. They audit for these higher charges on their patients' bills.

Previously, academic medicine argued it provided specialized services and higher quality care. This is no longer true. Nonprofits must compete with for-profit networks. This competition has forced academia to cut corners as well. They can no longer support and sustain their missions. In addition, they provide charity care. Charity patients use more resources than the average patient does. They do not access primary nor preventative care. Usually, these patients require emergency care for advanced illnesses, requiring extensive attention. These severe illnesses with their poor outcomes multiply the resources consumed.

Universal coverage is the best answer to the preservation of academic research and teaching. This is done by creating explicit, broad-based pools from all payers of health care. Together, everyone's premiums can collect volumes of interest. Quality medical education, biomedical and behavioral research, and the unique integrity of the not-for-profit mission is preserved. These centers are no match for cutthroat competition (Cohen, 1994). If academic medicine dies, everyone loses.

UNIVERSAL COVERAGE ELIMINATES HMOS

HMOs assume the least amount of risk amidst writing the rules of the game. Instead of physicians defining quality care, insurance executives are dictating efficient policy. Common sense would lead employers to deal directly with institutions, bypassing greedy middlemen. But cheaper administrative overhead, the power to streamline care, and pooling are advantages offered by middlemen. Giant managed care corporations can negotiate for volume discounts. Hospitals must agree to these discounts or lose thousands of patients. In turn, trimmed hospital budgets lead to poor patient satisfaction.

The incremental health care reform steps taken by Congress have encouraged this erosion. As these incremental steps have failed, the time for comprehensive reform has come. *The present model outline is that all profits go to the insurance industry, and all risk goes to providers and hospitals.* Congress could remove HMOs with antitrust legislation, and allow those with the risk to keep the profits to provide actual health care.

UNIVERSAL COVERAGE ELIMINATES A TWO-TIERED SYSTEM

Competing viewpoints result in obvious conflict. Stakeholders are those who pay for and those who receive coverage. These have opposite agendas. And then there are stakeholders who make policy, but are immune to the rules they make. They receive a higher tier of care as VIPs than the common patient. With universal coverage, private spending for health care is illegal. Those who make the policy get what everyone else gets. HMOs are eliminated.

UNIVERSAL COVERAGE EMPHASIZES PREVENTION

Presently, there is a conflict of interest with employers buying your care from HMOs. These folks are responsible for employees' health care. But they are looking out for their financial best interest.

Their contracts exist for an average of two years. How is your doctor to get to know you in two years? How does prevention occur in two years? What happens to treatment costs between plans? Remember, employees are productive, and therefore, healthy. But when employers have employees that use too much health care, the contract is dumped. Then, you must start over with a new doctor. HMOs want to provide the least amount of coverage—with preexisting condition clauses—for the most amount of an employer's money. Although they say prevention occurs in theory, in practice it is not a priority when plans change every two years. If the pool of employees becomes too risky or costly, the contract is not renewed and shopping for new contracts occurs. Employees are dumped when they really need their health care. But this is the purpose of getting benefits, so when you need health care you have it. HMOs are sending a different message: You must pay for health care, but you are not allowed to use it.

On employee retirement, the government provides Medicare. The retirement decades are ripe for chronic health problems. And illnesses are costly, exacerbated by years without preventative care. The government is content in shouldering this burden. This is counterintuitive because of the growing expenses incurred by the growing elderly population.

Insurers should be responsible for life spans of coverage. Then, preventative medicine would be built-in. Planning for wellness would be a true priority, rather than rhetoric. With universal coverage, the government is responsible for lifetimes of care. You would see monumental efforts channeled in this direction.

In addition to loss of freedom to choose providers and institutions, patients lose continuity of care and the prevention that goes with a provider who knows you well. Ignoring long-term healthy habits is encouraged by allowing HMOs to continue.

WHAT DOES THE CONSTITUTION AND THE CURRENT BILL OF RIGHTS SAY?

At this time, the U.S. and South Africa are the only countries that do not have universal health care coverage (Skolnick, 1996). The U.S. Constitution is silent on the issue of right to care. Only the mention of life, liberty, and the pursuit of happiness appears (neglected was the right to die issue). The Bill of Rights also neglects the health care issue. The exception is the Ninth Amendment which states that the listing of certain rights in the Constitution cannot be construed to deny others. The right to use birth control and abortion may be inferred, but actual access or care coverage is not defined as a right. Perhaps our founding fathers realized the complications inherent in establishing strict guidelines, and wisely chose not to pursue these avenues.

UNIVERSAL COVERAGE HARMS STATES

If socialized medicine were instituted, states would suffer. States are in better positions to recognize the needs of their habitants, and decentralization allows them the freedom to target relief. Rooted in the principles of classical federalism, policy makers in close proximity to constituents are best able to allocate resources effectively. But do emotional attachments lead to logical decision-making? Not always; major decisions about programs and populations are less subjective when decision-makers are removed from direct observation (Justice, 1995). What does this mean? Restated, decisions about *dollar* amounts should be federal decisions. State responsibilities should be needs assessments, methods to redistribute providers, rights and regulation enforcement, outcome measures, and feedback.

UNIVERSAL COVERAGE ESTABLISHES A NATIONAL DATA BANK

Some argue that socialized medicine has the advantage of a health system data bank, essential in implementing public health care delivery and subsequent policy. The Department of Health and Human Services (DHHS) is responsible for monitoring health care costs and their rates of increase.

With universal coverage, the DHHS would have complete and accurate access to condition-specific information and other areas, such as patient satisfaction (Greenfield, 1996). To those who favor universal coverage, this is occurring through the NCQA, who is collecting HEDIS outcomes.

UNIVERSAL COVERAGE DISADVANTAGES

Again, to adopt universal coverage would be to adopt the Canadian system and all its flaws. Socialized medicine means queuing, spending limitations per consumer, and maximum length of life issues. With universal coverage, patients have rights to advanced information without gag laws. However, private fund-raising or added insurance is not an option. Having more information is added torture when it is illegal to find a creative solution. An imperfect system will exist in this model, but then consider what we have now. Judgments are imposed on who can get an organ transplant. HMOs impose gag laws or "conscience clauses." There is no choice. Gatekeeping results in delays or refusals to refer, rigid and unreasonable rules of access. HMOs refuse to pay without obtaining prior permission.

This *unethical* rationing and ineligibility because of "preexisting conditions" is outright discrimination. What are the waiting differences between socialized medicine queuing and HMO referral waits? Things look similar in both cases. If socialized medicine replaces managed care discrimination and unethical rationing, which model is truly more limiting?

CONCLUSION

Which alternative does the greatest good for the most people? Your answer will depend if you are a patient, a provider, an HMO, a hospital, or other stakeholder listed in the box.

Each solution has advantages and disadvantages. What is the answer? Personally, I don't know. I have an opinion. If you read between the lines, you see I lean toward the consumer, primarily, and capitalism, secondarily. But just having an opinion does not make it right. My knowledge gives me no special expertise on this issue. No answer will be right for everyone.

References

Brostoff, Steven. (1993). "Majority Would Pay Tax for Universal Coverage: Poll." *National Underwriter Life & Health-Financial Services Edition* (18), 34.

Cohen, Jordan. (1994). "Why Is Academic Medicine Dying for Universal Coverage?" *American Medical News 37* (31), 23.

Deloitte & Touche LLP. (11-13-98). Trim: A Newsletter for the Healthcare Field.

Fulton, Jane. (1994). Keynote address representing University of Ottawa Strategic Management and Ethics. The Annual Risk and Insurance Management Society Conference.

Greenfield, Lee. (1996). "Without Universal Coverage, Health Care Use Data Do Not Provide Population Health." *The Milbank Quarterly 74* (1), 33.

Justice, Diane. (Fall, 1995). "The Aging Network: A Balancing Act Between Universal Coverage and Defined Eligibility." *Generations 19* (3), 58.

Kenkel, Paul. (1994). "Minnesota Officials Want to Delay Network Start." *Modern Healthcare 24* (9), 3.

Klass, Perri. (10-5-97). "Managing Managed Care." *The New York Times Magazine.*

McDermott, James. (1995). "The First Step. (Universal Coverage Is Foundation for Health Care Reform)." *JAMA 273,* (3), 251.

McIllrath, Sharon. (1994). "Ways & Means Calls for Universal Coverage, Employer Mandate." *American Medical News 37,* (27), 3.

Merriam-Webster. (1989). *The New Merriam-Webster Dictionary.* Merriam-Webster: Springfield, Massachusetts.

Monahan, P. (7-15-98). Caring for Medicare. *The Globe and Mail.*

National Public Radio Broadcast. (April 1997). California Physicians Take On Managed Care. Denver, CO.

Skolnick, Andrew. (1996). "Democrats Drop Universal Coverage." *JAMA 276,* (12), 931.

Reinhardt, Uwe. (8-1-96). "Will Physicians Take Back Medicine?" *Physician Executive.*

Tenery, Robert M. Jr. (1994). "Don't Confuse Universal Access with Universal Coverage." *American Medical News 37,* (18), 30.

Voelker, Rebecca. (1993). "Is Reform Coverage Really Universal?" *JAMA 270,* (22), 2663.

Wyke, Alexandra. (July/August, 1997). "Can Patients Drive the Future of Health Care?" *Harvard Business Review.*

CHAPTER 13

What Happens as Things Change?

Managed care takes credit for being the change agent for modern innovation. Yes, many positive things are occurring. But, here are some side effects of managed care. And there are far-reaching implications.

MERGERS AND ACQUISITIONS

Mergers and acquisitions reduce costs—and quality. It is difficult to pick up a newspaper and not read about some merger or acquisition. In any industry, having a simple cost structure or one set of expenses reduces overhead. One team can run several HMOs rather than several teams of high salaried officers run one. But the most important advantage of acquiring other HMOs is acquiring "lives." The more covered lives an HMO has, the more power it has. Hospitals and provider groups will promise larger discounts to HMOs who can guarantee patients needing services. But as hospitals and providers try to meet their discounts, they cut corners. The art to healing is forgotten. There is little time for listening. Rather than humans, patients become "encounters." Something projected or forecasted for HMO growth. Today's leaders are afraid of changing this because this money saved is money taxed. Money saved supports campaigns. The more businesses grow, the more the customer is taken for granted. But dissatisfied customers cannot return "products" in health care. With surgery and certain procedures, all sales are final.

▲ 125

PREVENTION

Prevention enters the equation—for some. Mind-sets were supposed to change. Entry into the health care system should move away from the hospitalization event. Prevention is to become the standard with managed care. This is based on the penny-wise and pound-foolish cliché. It is cheaper to maintain health over time than to invest in rebuilding crashing organs or futile tissue. The theory of capitation was prepaid health care. HMOs pay providers to keep their patients healthy, hence the name, health maintenance organizations. Doctors use disease management techniques to *prevent* rather than be ruled by illness. This occurs from birth to death. Examples are giving immunizations to the young and walkers to the old to prevent fractured hips. The National Institute for Health is funding clinical research for relaxation, aerobics, and dietary counseling.

But greed tarnishes good intentions. In practice, whose health is being maintained? HMOs only want young and healthy patients. Healthy patients can work. And their employers *pay* their health premiums. Therefore, it is better to keep patients healthy so they can work. Employees create rather than consume cash flows. Where does this leave the rest of us?

CONSUMER AWARENESS

Protocols and pathways are becoming a built-in medical record, based on real time. These critical pathways are tomorrow's form of Total Quality Management (TQM). New "Clinical Guidelines," best care practices, and treatment schedules are published everywhere you look. Cookbook medicine will drive health care, rather than individualism. The disadvantage to using protocols for severe illnesses is everyone becomes an expert. Decisions will be made based on health care "bibles," not common sense. The wrong people end up making choices for you.

On-line and multimedia raises the bar for patients' education. Decision support systems assist in difficult or ethical dilemmas. On-call media may even replace "Ask a Nurse" call systems. As consumers become educated, we may see a voucher system. Your employer or the state will disburse medical care allotments and you choose your own health care benefits.

Integrated delivery systems will encompass employers and communities. In fact, your network may begin at your workplace or community. The advantage to relaxing the institutional mindset is returning a proper focus on community health concerns. More money is spent specific to community needs. Disadvantages are how to handle common data pool battles, turf issues, and confidentiality of information.

DISEASE MANAGEMENT

When diagnoses acquire price tags, attention can be paid to the most expensive diagnoses affecting the most people. The three biggest costs identified are: high-risk pregnancy, workers' compensation, and wellness. This means if your particular illness is not popular, expect less attention in health care. Resources will be shifted from overused low-value disease treatments to underused high-value practices. Rather than concentrating on premiums and profits, concern turns to what drives the costs of medical care.

ASSISTED LIVING

Medicare and Medicaid waivers allow competition to replace previous socialized medicine. This allows states to sell groups of government patients to HMOs. The HMOs provide more efficient care by getting their discounts for large numbers. As the elderly population increases, nursing home costs will become astronomical. Now is the time to establish assisted living communities based on the waiver system.

But no HMO wants these types of patients. Therefore, some states are assigning a proportionate share of these patients to each HMO. If an HMO wants a license to operate, the state mandates participation in care for government patients. If not, licenses are revoked. One side effect is that HMOs are beginning to declare Chapter 11 bankruptcy.

TOO MUCH CHANGE TOO FAST

Patients seem frustrated by the pace and the pressures of change in modern health care. It is difficult to cope when decisions are made without the input of the majority. When you or a loved one's health is in concern, there is stress. When the rules change for each provider visit, there is anger, blame, and frustration.

Too much change has blown constituents out of the water. Leaders need to shift some of the control back to the people. The uncertainly is uncomfortable. However, people seem ready to vote for some major relief.

ALTERNATIVE THERAPIES

Politics in medicine has created barriers for unconventional healing methods. These barriers breed secrecy in patients searching for alternate modalities and spiritual enrichment. What does the medical world offer the human dimension but the fifteen-minute office visit? Medicine is not a transpersonal business for recharging batteries. The growing availability and success of other methods suggests an increased resistance toward the rigidly defined patient role, a role that is unnatural, unsatisfying, and incomplete.

The medical model is disease-oriented. An intense focus on epidemiology occupies one end of the spectrum. In the medical model, the mind is separated from the body. Treating physical diseases is the main priority. This is a powerful, profound, and necessary mission. How does one heal the mind? If medicine is unable to provide a total package, this omission should be acknowledged, and credence given to complementary therapies. A balanced view is not used to promote healing of the mind and body with managed care.

If biologic, chemical, or alternative interventions offer relief, therein lies the answer. Some disease processes are not fully understood by the champions of science. Therefore, is it a patient's right to seek more knowledge? Providers are held to invoke the ethical principle of non-maleficence, or do no harm. Treatments should not conflict, and complete honesty is necessary with all providers. Large doses of herbs or megavitamin regimes may interfere with lab results and interact with prescribed medications. Common sense must prevail in using complementary approaches such as acupuncture, chiropractic, naturopathy, homeopathy, osteopathy, and others. Modern practitioners should work with sufferers of chronic pain to find better methods of relief. Unfortunately, there are few if any managed care protocols that address alternative solutions.

A good medical doctor will never dismiss therapies that offer safe relief and healing of the mind and body. All disciplines have something to offer and must work together when patients solicit help from varied sources. Partnerships must form between those who excel in areas of alternative care—partnerships that treat the whole patient with complementary rather than duplicated services. There will be more money available if overlapped or disconnected care is eliminated. We must not allow care to become streamlined to where mental health and psychological concerns are ignored. Currently, our society fails to address social problems until they become medical problems. Examples are substance abuse, domestic violence, and child abuse. Our next system must be designed to restore patients' trust in the medical industry. Therapies must be built into the network to maintain the welfare of society.

CONCLUSION

Health care will not be chaotic forever. The leaders of society and organizations with sound strategies for quality care will be the ones standing when the dust settles. For now, it is a matter of finding out who they are and voting them into office.

References

Lumsdom, K. (November, 1996). "Executives of Seven Large Health Care Companies Discuss Changes in Health Care Systems. *Hospitals and Health Networks.*

Zaher, C. (1996). Learning to Be a Leader. *Physician Executive 22,* (10).

CHAPTER 14

How Will Managed Care Hurt Progress?

"Evil does not prevail everywhere. But to ignore evil is to blind oneself to reality."
—Henry David Thoreau

WINNERS AND LOSERS

To ignore the evils of managed care is to blind ourselves to many realities. HMOs have millions of dollars in assets. HMO CEOs make as much money as basketball players when stock options are exercised. This is the reward for instituting efficient health care. Investor-owned HMOs cater to their stockholders rather than their covered lives. To create dividends, HMOs will not pay for treatments that stop disease and death if they are not cost-effective. But, the methods they use to determine cost-effectiveness may discriminate against you.

Health care coverage is not a necessity. Food, water, shelter, and the means to provide these things are. Health policies are a luxury. This type of health care luxury has opportunity costs. Besides feeding HMOs your hard-earned money through your employer, HMOs cost you in other ways.

▲ Loss of freedom to change plans. Changing to cheaper plans interrupts continuity of care. Patients fall between the cracks when treatments are interrupted.

▲ HMOs create society costs. Rather than buy managed care, some opt for no health care for more salary. This creates costs to society in the long run.

▲ Loss of a public good. (See page 139.)

Why are you paying so much to an HMO that gives so little in return? They do not pay for treatments that stop all disease and death, only the ones that don't cost them money. Money is not the only measure of cost-effectiveness.

OTHER WAYS TO MEASURE EFFECTIVENESS

J. Bean (1994) shares another way managed care hurts progress.

"The president of a large California managed care company was also chairman of the board of his community's symphony orchestra. Finding he could not go to one of the concerts, he gave his tickets to the company's director of health care cost containment. The next morning, he asked the director how he enjoyed the performance. Instead of the expected usual polite remarks, the director handed him a memo which read as follows.

The undersigned submits the following comments and recommendations relative to the performance of Schubert's Unfinished Symphony by the Civic Orchestra as observed under actual working conditions:

▲ *The attendance of the orchestra conductor is unnecessary for public performances. The orchestra has obviously practiced and has the prior authorization from the conductor to play the symphony at a predetermined level of quality. Considerable money could be saved by merely having the conductor critique the orchestra's performance during a retrospective peer review meeting.*

▲ *For considerable periods, the four oboe players had nothing to do. Their numbers should be reduced and their work spread over the whole orchestra, thus eliminating peaks and valleys of activity.*

▲ *All 12 violins were playing identical notes with identical motions. This is unnecessary duplication; the staff of this section should be drastically cut with consequent savings. If a large volume of sound is required, this could be obtained through electronic amplification, which has reached high levels of reproductive quality.*

▲ *Much effort was expended playing 16th notes, or semi-quavers. This seems an excessive refinement as most of the listeners are unable to distinguish such rapid playing. It is recommended that all notes be rounded up to the nearest 8th. If this is done, it would be possible to use trainees and lower grade operators with no loss of quality.*

▲ *No useful purpose would appear to be served by repeating with horns the same passage that has already been handled by the strings. If all such redundant passages were eliminated, as determined by the utilization review committee, the concert could have been reduced from two hours to 20 minutes, with greater savings in salaries and overhead. In fact, if Schubert had attended to these matters on a cost containment basis, he probably would have been able to finish his symphony."*

DESIGNER DRUGS: STATINS AND VIAGRA

Statins lower cholesterol and prevent heart disease. Drug companies argue if heart disease is the number one cause of death, the majority of Americans should take statins. Another designer drug is Viagra, which resolves impotence. Both these drugs are marketed directly to the public. This encourages more moral hazard. If someone else pays, everyone wants designer drugs. But some plans refuse to pay for new and expensive drugs for everyone. There is long-term evidence to support use of statins for high-risk patients only. And both Viagra and statins have many side effects. One side effect of Viagra is pregnancy. Some argue why should Viagra be free and birth control not? The floodgates could open. Who should pay for fertility treatments?

WHO GETS DESIGNER DRUGS?

HMOs decide. They have guidelines allowing high-risk persons to take statins. You get statins only if you have high cholesterol. High cholesterol is defined as a blood chemistry value of over 240 units. Some literature advocates treating patients with a cholesterol of 180, if they have elevated low density lipid (LDL) values. This issue provokes many ethical and technological controversies surrounding designer drugs, another issue where health care is not black and white. HMO guidelines are based on cost-effective analyses (CEA). But there are flaws in CEA formulas when opportunity and social costs are not included.

COSTS OF DESIGNER DRUGS IN HEALTH CARE

The costs of using statins are measured in dollars. The costs of *not* using statins cannot be measured in dollars. They are measured in higher cholesterol levels and more heart disease. With the current lack of patients' rights, you cannot sue your HMO to be on statins.

COST-EFFECTIVE ANALYSES

CEA is a collection of methods used to prioritize and allocate resources. This maximizes desirable outcomes. The idea came from public project priority setting such as funding dams, parks, and highways. When CEA techniques are applied to medicine, it creates values for treatments. When the worth of treatments are known, they may be prioritized and rationed. Highest priority are given to the treatments that provide the greatest benefit per cost.

The formula for a cost-effective ratio is: costs/benefits. Costs are defined in dollars. And benefits are defined in units of: QALY (Quality Adjust Life Years) or HBUs (Health Benefit Units). Then, these steps are followed.

1. *Benefits or outcomes are estimated for each treatment.*
2. *Costs are estimated for each treatment.*
3. *Dividing the two tells how greatly treatment costs cut into treatment benefits.*
4. *If a treatment's costs are too much for benefits received, it receives no priority.*

When HMOs have a limited budget, they may decide to pay for the top ten or twenty treatments that are most cost-effective (Eddy, 1992).

HMOs are not responsible to provide every new technology to every patient.

This same situation surfaces each time a new drug emerges. Drug companies market a biased view. Patients ask physicians to prescribe these therapies. Drug companies who attempt to educate the public need to give broader information. These drugs are not right for everyone. All medications, including statins, have side effects. Statins can cause harm to the liver or heart muscle.

Intestinal problems, liver, and heart damage may lead to expensive ER visits.

Physicians, not HMOs, should determine cases individually. When doctors prescribe statins, they take on added monitoring responsibilities. Starting patients on these drugs or changing dosages means blood must be drawn at intervals to check blood chemistries. These are added costs for monitoring patients on sensitive drugs. Physicians are busy people. They know that every choice involves opportunity costs. More time and resources are spent on a few. This means less of their time and resources for other patients.

CONSUMER SOVEREIGNTY

What if each person placed a value on life? How much are you willing to pay for treatments that keep you alive? With MSAs, consumers could decide which treatments are best. But veto power must be returned to physicians from HMOs guidelines.

- ▲ Consumer decisions may be irrational, and ignore side effects. Taking statins is not a license to practice an unhealthy lifestyle. Statins represent a lazy way to lower cholesterol rather than exercising or maintaining a fat restricted diet. Purchases of Viagra may be at the expense of another family member's blood pressure medication.

- ▲ Patients on statins are told not to smoke or drink, but continue to do so. Resistance to medical advice raises a red flag. Patients who are noncompliant in one area may be so in many. Noncompliant patients may not show for frequent blood draws and other monitors. This is a cost to others who might have used these scarce resources.

- ▲ The consumer is not the best nor the only judge to determine risk factors for a heart attack. Similarly, the consumer should not be the sole decision-maker of how to treat a high cholesterol level. Most patients will do better with a low fat intake and exercise. This involves no blood draws, monitoring costs, or side effects.

Providers, and then consumers, should have the most power in deciding how to allocate scarce resources. This position advocates medical paternalism. However, physicians, and not patients or HMOs, are the ones with the most knowledge about how drugs work and patients' situations. Physicians have the best perspective of who is helped with statins. They will make the most rational decisions in the treatment of hypercholesterolemia. With providers' input, patients may self-ration.

CONCEPTUAL FLAWS IN CEA

Cost-Effectiveness Analyses (CEA) are the favored method for rationing therapies and guiding practices. The biggest problem occurs before formulas are applied. The numbers plugged into these formulas are estimates. QALYs and HBUs are arbitrary. Although these formulas are padded for error, they decide life and death prognoses. HMO economists are able to be distant and calculate who gets what services. But who delivers the bad news—providers. Some health care economists consider providers to be too involved. Often, they are not invited to help determine rationing benefits. Providers have all the responsibility, but none of the power. These inconsistencies prove providers should be more involved in rationing decisions.

▲ Tooth caps are cheap and provide more long-term benefits. This has a higher priority than surgical removal of an ectopic pregnancy. Although the latter saves a life, it is not cost-effective. Death, an opportunity cost, is not figured into CEAs.

- Autologous bone marrow transplants are not cost-effective, yet screens for cancer are. If cancer treatments are denied, why do HMOs pay for testing?
- Rare and unusual diseases are biased from the start, due to learning curve costs.
- Diseases in children are weighted more heavily than for the elderly. This is discrimination. How do children provide more social value than the older, educated, and more experienced?
- How are multiple diagnoses or benefit factors combined in this formula?
- Initially, kidney transplants were not cost-effective when compared to hemodialysis. Now, a kidney transplant is cheaper than maintaining patient on hemodialysis.
- The cost of overhead is ignored in CEA. Fixed costs such as equipment, heat, mortgages or rent, technology, and others, are not a part of formulas' cost.
- Practices are not steady over time. What was previously done as inpatient is now outpatient. What is done as an outpatient today may become a home health treatment tomorrow. Costs for some expensive treatments are going down. They are becoming more affordable. These lags will not show up in CEA tables for years. By then, it will be too late for some HMO patients. And some HMOs cannot be sued.
- Since it is impossible to define economic or opportunity costs, accounting costs are used. Accounting costs are estimated, and they depend on an institution's volume and discretion. Also, these costs reflect the creativity of an accountant. These costs are not comparable globally.

▲ Social value is ignored. Dollar benefits have higher value than the benefits that humans provide.

Whose definition is used to decide what treatments have more benefits than others? What is used as a biological basis for cost and benefit? These concepts mean different things to an accountant, to a cancer biologist, to you, or to me. But economists are doing this and claiming success at it. CEA is not an ironclad method for prioritizing benefits. CEA is a smokescreen for cutting treatments for those with expensive diseases. Current priorities are angina, gallstones, hip arthritis, uterine conditions, and prostate conditions (Wennberg, J., 10-25-90). If your diagnosis is not here, you are paying you HMO to discriminate against you.

THE LOSS OF A PUBLIC GOOD

Reducing contagious diseases is not a concern of managed care. For example, few HMOs find covering HIV treatments profitable. This is another complex reason why health care is not a normal market. A public good is a good in which all of society benefits equally. When one consumer shares in a public good, others' shares are not diminished. Examples are public defense, research knowledge, and satellite technology.

Since health care is a corporate-run market, no one will produce public goods. The cost of these advantages is small in industrialized countries. If they offer a bigger bang for the buck, why don't we spend more on them? But with managed care no one profits from producing public goods, so no one does. The government is the one entity that forces people to pay for public goods through taxation. HMOs could pay a public good tax to support the costs of public good innovation, research to control contagious diseases, and other nonprofitable technologies.

Meanwhile, HMOs remain free riders when others shoulder learning curve costs.

OTHER FACTORS THAT CONSTRAIN COSTS

▲ *Direct Costs: Bureaucratic red tape that slows or inhibits reimbursement, legislative constraints that favor businesses against patients, political parties' campaign financing, gatekeeping, inflated demand.*

▲ *Indirect Costs: Legal costs to defend providers and insurers, career entry issues such as restrictive licensing, unions that demand quality benefits, persons with short-term goals, no conscience for long-term survival of quality institutions.*

▲ *Social Costs: Pollution, tobacco, drug, or alcohol habits at the expense of the family unit, non-compliant patients who refuse to follow their treatment.*

▲ *Opportunity Costs: Time lost waiting to see providers, healing time lost by foregoing a better health care option, preventable deaths.*

ECONOMIC MALPRACTICE

It is difficult to achieve economic efficiency when managing scarce resources. In the statin case, rationing occurs better through providers than HMOs. If HMO guidelines are mandated to providers, even guidelines need guidelines. Guidelines are not and should not be absolutes. Flexibility must be built into protocols. It is in the best interest of science to continually question standards set by humans. This proves physicians, not HMOs, must be involved in making rationing policy. Providers must be allowed to decide cases individually.

Yes, economic experts need to make economic recommendations. But ultimately, health care decisions should be influenced by experts in health care. Flawed or incomplete CEA data is not acceptable for basing medical practice. Nor should it be accepted for rationing policy. It is irresponsible to use information that is— of questionable validity, subject to interpretation, or too technical for laypersons to understand—to dominate resource allocation.

CEA is helpful in arbitrarily prioritizing treatment by dollars spent. But it is too difficult to compute true costs or true benefits. The definitions of both "cost" and "benefit" involve more abstract than concrete units. It is impossible to force the laws of nature to conform to business principles. Too many variables are removed and ignored in order to create an artificial, simplistic means of discrimination. When the world shares its complicated but crucial facts and constants, we should offer thanks for such a boost to understanding. (Gould, 1996).

References

Bean, J. (8-19-94). *Psychiatric News Issue.* San Francisco, CA: APA.

Eddy, D. (1992). "Cost-Effective Analysis: A Conversation with My Father." *JAMA 267,* (3), 1669– 1675.

Eddy, D. (1992). "Applying Cost Effective Analysis: The Inside Story." *JAMA 268,* (18), 2575–2582.

Gould, S. (1996). *The Mismeasure of Man.* New York, NY: W. W. Norton & Company.

Hildred, W. & Watkins L. (1996). "The Nearly Good, the Bad, and the Ugly in Cost-Effectiveness Analysis of Health Care." *The Journal of Economic Issues.*

Wennberg, J. (10-25-90). "Outcomes Research: Cost-Containment and the Fear of Health Care Rationing." *NEJM 323,* (21), 1202.

CHAPTER 15

So What Happens Next?

What Does the Future Hold?

In his book *Megatrends*, John Naisbitt predicts the following changes in health care.

▲ Information technology is more important than industrialization.

▲ Values are changing toward convenience and quality of life issues.

▲ Cost constraints will spawn new models and settings for health care.

▲ Consumers demand accountability.

To see if he is right, we will examine how each prediction has evolved. Then we will examine more predictions about the health care of tomorrow.

INFORMATION TECHNOLOGY

This is the key to establishing integrated delivery systems. If the clinic to hospital to home care model is to become seamless, the clinic provider must have the same information that the last hospital nurse or home health care nurse records. You should not have to recreate your last medical encounter. This will eliminate health care professionals playing detective. Reasons why you were started on a new drug should be available in a database. Videoconferencing for consultations or second opinions makes diagnosing more accurate. Radio waves and cell phone connections have enabled communication to occur in real time. Patient education involves virtual reality or interactive kiosks.

Change runs a rampant pace in the computer industry. Health care mirrors this industry due to its dependence on computer technology. So how does the computer world do strategic planning? And how might this affect health care strategic planning? Too much is changing too fast. Previously, success was defined by how responsive a business was to customer demand. Now, it is not enough to be responsive. Success is predicting what the customer wants before (s)he knows what it is. In health care, consumerism makes these predictions easy. Whoever gives consumers what they want can retire early.

CONVENIENCE IN HEALTH CARE

Americans are demanding more convenience in health care. Payers of health care want more home health and outpatient services. Combining the two is easily done.

Outpatient centers must appeal to the consumer with juice bars, playgrounds, and exercise clubs. Traffic areas, soft space, and buffer zones should be designed around two settings: inpatient and outpatient facilities. A serious inpatient setting and a softer outpatient setting should be split by shared ancillary disciplines. Fiber-optic capability is shared.

Why not place mini-malls in these centers' halls? Crane (1993) in *Professional Services Marketing* tells us to locate ourselves in areas where consumers do multiple errands. Why not bring the shops to the consumer? Move main floor offices to unused bed space and lease prime ground floor space? One of the biggest complaints is long waiting times. Supply beepers or install an overhead paging system encouraging patients to shop. Provide kiosks, patient education videos, or pamphlets for those who prefer to sit. What about waiting room lending libraries? Nordstrom's offers mammograms for women shoppers.

Satellite centers such as rehab, ophthalmology, or physical therapy are also set up in communities—away from the hospital atmosphere, accessible, and leased rather than built.

QUALITY OF LIFE ISSUES

Americans are demanding more emphasis on quality of life in health care. To a certain extent this is an emphasis on ethics. Ethics are moral principles governing human conduct. Moral principles concern what ought to be done and why. Law is always subject to change because laws are based on society's values. Society's values change over time, and laws follow the values of society. If this is true, how do we answer these questions for the future?

▲ What role does the law play in morality? Are we too dependent on the law? Is law the working source of morality?

▲ There is more competition and ethical claims are met with rationing. If all lives are of equal worth, how do we allocate treatments? Conversely, if we believe some lives are "worth" more, then how is worthiness decided?

▲ What duty do we have to protect the weak? What duty do we have to preserve life? What does loyalty to patients require?

▲ What are concepts of life and death and what are legal standards? What are criteria to determining who is "alive" or dead? And to what extent do/should we err on the side of inclusion regarding life?

▲ Should ethical questions or morality be based on rights or duty?

▲ If moral questions have societal consequences, and there are moral truths that are absolute, to what extent are we doing things not because we have moral/ethical grounding, but rather because we have the ability (cloning)?

▲ We know that health care cannot promise cure. We know that health care cannot promise to relieve suffering. What can health care promise—only to be present. If this is true, then what is presence? Do we need to look beyond medical models for presence?

We, as a society, cannot answer these questions. But we, as individuals, can. Laws will not and cannot address each topic fairly. But if consumers are allowed to self-ration, these questions can be defined and answered by individuals.

CONSUMERS DEMAND ACCOUNTABILITY

You are in the hospital. Your HMO protocol says it is time for you to go home. But your body is not following the protocol rules. How will you get your doctor to agree to invest more hospital time and resources into keeping you hospitalized? Does everyone have the chance to be as healthy as anyone else? The ethical principles of justice and non-maleficence may be justification for more care. It is a myth that the average amount of care for a given diagnosis is the ideal amount of care. Imagine a plot of costs over time of a million patients' hospital course with your same problem. A normal bell-shaped curve would appear. There will be some who consume more and some who consume less. Patients will not be treated fairly if too few or too many resources are committed to them. But how can we do the most good with the limited resources available, and who receives the benefits? By determining where you fit on the bell curve, your care can be adjusted to reflect an ethically acceptable portion of care that you need.

What if you have a MSA? You will want to go home so as not to empty your account. Ask your doctor or case manager to arrange care at home. Do you see how moral hazard works? Do you see how shifting power back to the consumer changes how health care is consumed?

COST CONSTRAINTS SPAWN NEW MODELS

Although most providers are great people, you should not trust everything they say. I am not in favor of letting physicians make my decisions for me. I want to spend my health care dollars in the way I think is most beneficial to my needs. I don't believe that I am alone in this feeling.

What if your doctor wants to do major surgery on your back when you would rather see a chiropractor and/or try simple medication? Doctors overvalue medicine just as military officers overvalue defense spending. The well-meaning physician may wrongly conclude that extensive care is required when simple care could do more good and less harm. A physician's definition of a benefit is different than yours or mine. When it is impossible for physicians and patients to articulate true agendas, patients buy into a demand for more care. Patients have many concerns: social, economic, aesthetic, spiritual, organic, and psychological. Patients have values and beliefs that are different from the medical community's. A physician must be omniscient to prescribe the best treatment for you. Providers do not know which interventions are most beneficial.

By allowing patients to refuse or define their own care, autonomy is invoked and costs will be saved. The health care community of tomorrow must be allowed to grow around the true need of patients. This can only be defined by patients.

PREDICTIONS FOR THE FUTURE OF HEALTH CARE

- Universal coverage will not be accepted into our capitalistic society. If used correctly, competition favors patients. Big businesses may be rewarded with profit if they offer patients what they want.
- The welfare system will be decreased by workfare, but remain in some form. HMOs may be around to coordinate efficient care for elderly or poverty patients.
- Medicare will become extinct in our lifetime because of the aging baby boomers. Families will take more responsibility in addition to growth of assisted living programs.
- Academic institutions will become for-profit. Pharmaceutical companies will finance their innovative research. Education goes on-line (see below). Charity care is assumed by state-run HMOs.
- On-line college educations will increase the supply of doctors and nurses. Providers' salaries will go down if supply is increased and demand relaxes.
- MSAs will affect the middle to upper classes. Some limitations will evolve to protect MSA over-utilization. DRG limits or some new buzzword will protect from fee-for-service abuses. Other exploitations are prevented by for-profit agents and health care consultants.
- Demand management will evolve. Telephone 1-800-callnurse centers will triage your illness/injury by phone. While looking at your health and insurance records on-line, they will guide the best immediate action to be taken, guided by your health care coverage. If you choose to go to the ER anyway, you will pay the costs you incur. Managing health care demand is the rationale.

References

Alters. (1994). "The Myth of Long-Term Planning. *Computerworld.*

Anonymous. (1997). "Clinton Names Panel to Bolster Health Care Rights; Reforms: High-Level Commission Is to Develop Ways to Protect Patients and Assure Quality Treatment Under Managed Care Programs (Home Ed.)." *The Los Angeles Times.*

Anonymous. (1997). "Doctors: Cutting Back the Supply." *The New York Times.*

Anonymous. (1997). "Settlements: Tobacco, Cars, and Implants." *The New York Times.*

Bond, M., Hrivnak, M., & Heshizer, B. (1996). "Reducing Employee Health Expenses with Medical Savings Accounts." *Compensation & Benefits Review.*

Brock, R. (1996). "Head for Business: Managed Care Demands Business Savvy. Here's How Nurses Get It" (excerpt from book, *The Business of Nursing*). In *Hospitals & Health Networks.*

Conan, N., Silberner, J., Davidson, R., & Rothschild. (1994). "Health Care Reform to Rely Heavily on HMOs." *NPR* (morning edition).

Cornwell, S. (1997). "Clinton Names Commission to Monitor Health Care." *Reuters, Ltd.*

Crane, F. (1993). *Professional Services Marketing: Strategy and Tactics.* NY: The Haworth Press.

DeParle, J. (1997). "Getting Opal Caples to Work." *The New York Times Magazine.*

Dorgan, C. (1995). *Statistical Record of Health & Medicine.* New York, NY: Thompson Publishing Company.

Hildred, W., & Watkins, L. (1996). "The Nearly Good, the Bad, and the Ugly in Cost-Effectiveness Analysis of Health Care." *Journal of Economic Issues.*

Kenney. (1996). "Facilities Design in a Managed Care Environment." *Hospital Topics.*

MacPherson, P. (1996). "Agency Talk: Reports of the Health Care Financing Administration's Death Are Greatly Exaggerated." *Hospitals & Health Networks 70,* (3), 39.

Phelps, C. (1997). *Health Care Economics* (2nd Ed.). Menlo Park, CA: Addison-Wesley Educational Publishers, Inc.

Veatch, R. (1986). "DRGs and the Ethical Reallocation of Resources." *Hastings Center Report.*

Vickery, D. & Lynche W. (1995). "Demand Management: Enabling Patients to Use Medical Care Appropriately." *JOEM, 37,* (5), 1–7.

Whitman, D. & Cooper, M. (1996). "Fixing the Welfare Mess." *U.S. News & World Report.*

CHAPTER 16

What Are Your Rights?

"If the misery of our poor be caused not by the laws of nature, but by our institutions, great is our sin."
—Charles Darwin

The purpose of this book has been to outline the difficulties in changing health care. It is a big responsibility to balance equities and costs in health care. But I believe quality health care can be provided in a cost-effective manner. We all agree that major improvements are needed. But if the system is bent too far, it could break. Any small changes will increase health care costs. Higher deductibles, premiums, and co-payments will be used to finance the changes. But strict rights favoring patients too much are large changes that could force HMOs out of business. No one will be an HMO if they must provide first-class health care for no profits. Hospitals and providers must be allowed to make profits, also. If not, rational behavior kicks in. No one will practice medicine without incentives. A realistic compromise must occur by all.

Extreme measures such as fee-for-service proved unsuccessful. But is socialized medicine the answer? The Canadians don't think so. What is the answer? I don't know. I have an opinion, but it is neither right nor wrong. My hope is to lay out the situations, identify the stakeholders and their behaviors. I leave the rest up to you. With this vital information, perhaps you can identify a better way. And if enough of us put our heads together, we can make a difference.

A NEW HEALTH CARE BILL OF RIGHTS

You may believe that a bill of rights is the answer. You may have some rights already. You may live in a state that has high standards for HMOs. Currently, states are writing or passing bills to regulate managed care. These bills can be found on-line; however, they are difficult to interpret. They should attempt to address the following issues.

- ▲ Access to Health Care: Geographically specific terms must be identified to ensure that patients are provided appropriate high-quality care.
- ▲ Access to Clinical Trials: Who pays and how much is contributed for experimentation.
- ▲ Appeals: Bad medicine cannot be encouraged, nor can overcompensatory rewards. However, consumers need a mechanism to resolve their differences with health plans and health care providers.
- ▲ At-risk populations: Alternate therapies for high-risk persons to find relief must be allowed. Language to punish discrimination is needed.
- ▲ Compliance: Everyone shares in accountability.
- ▲ Consumer Choice and Responsibility: Patients must have the tools to reward excellent providers.
- ▲ Disclosure of Information: Informed consent is necessary to make life and death decisions
- ▲ Emergency Service: Guidelines are needed to define "emergency," and steps to be followed when and where the need arises.
- ▲ Enforcement: Establish a mechanism for audits and penalties for any stakeholder who breaches his responsibility.

- ▲ Financial Disincentives: Incentives must be removed from providers to prevent patient harm. This must include failure to refer, bonuses, utilization, and other conflicts of interest.
- ▲ Pharmacy Formularies: There must be ways to get around limits in medication lists.
- ▲ Quality of Care: Universal protocols must be established for a minimum of care.

Some states have crude, but commendable starts in drafting health care rights. The problem is how to define the above terms. No one definition will match the definition of all perspectives. Your legislators know this. Perhaps you can write and give your legislators some help. But first, some background in the task of writing regulations.

THE THEORY OF REGULATION

There are two kinds of regulations (Stigler, 1971). One protects and benefits the public. The other creates a means to a political end. A virtuous example of the latter is when the slaves were free. A vulgar example is unnecessary salary raises that feather Congressional nests. Because of this power, the federal or state systems are machines. Machines that redistribute wealth are trading power in certain ways:

- ▲ to design motives that prohibit or compel,
- ▲ to take away or give money, and
- ▲ to help or hurt parties involved in the health care industry.

Ways to Regulate Supply

▲ *A tax on a powerful industry is a disincentive which slows supply.*

▲ *Give subsidies to weaker industries to encourage business.*

▲ *Control entry of new arrivals with strict or relaxed licensing.*

▲ *Provide substitutes such as nurse practitioners to encourage access.*

▲ *Price-fixing is another disincentive which slows supply.*

▲ *Antitrust Regulation. This is already in place. But state waivers allow and encourage HMOs to contain costs. State waivers could be revoked, though unlikely, as no back-up plan exists.*

▲ *Industry Survival Regulation. This may be needed to fund future medical practices if too many providers leave.*

▲ *Community Survival Regulation. The definition of community could include the elderly or poverty populations. An example of this regulation is reimbursing nurse practitioners for treating Medicare patients. This safeguards certain populations.*

Health care supply is scarce and the demand is inflated. Your state or the federal government could limit supply by setting prices. But there are disadvantages to price fixing in a growing economy. A better way might be to limit competition between HMOs. This can be done through licensing. States can control the number of HMOs by granting or withholding licenses. This could prevent new HMOs from entering your region and lowering prices or care standards. States can raise or lower licensing standards, also. This is how states can enforce patients' rights.

But if HMOs are insulted too much, they will go elsewhere. To entice them, states pay subsidies to HMOs to care for high-risk patients. So you see, states need HMOs as much as they need taxpayers.

WHO SHOULD RATION YOUR CARE?

Britain and Canada ration health care. They spend less money per patient per year than the United States does. Who has the healthiest population? They share similar outcomes in morbidity and mortality as we do (Phelps, 1997). This leads to the conclusion that rationing does not lead to bad outcomes. Many of our fancy or expensive treatments are not worthwhile. We throw more money at futile problems, and this is why HMOs may be around a while. They are turning health care costs around.

Like it or not, we must get used to the idea of rationing. But we should have more control in how it is done. This is America, and we are a different breed. Let Canada and the UK be content with socialized medicine, but let us ration on our own terms. If we must ration, let us decide how and where our premiums are spent.

You may believe that Medical Savings Accounts or a related concept is the answer. If you believe you should control your health care dollars and decisions, tell your legislators.

The Internet addresses for the House and Senate are as follows:

http://www.house.gov
http://www.senate.gov

COMING FULL CIRCLE: CONSUMERISM

This book started with consumerism, and it ends with consumerism. I could take more time to write, but it is time to stop. Your time is valuable and could be used in another important way—to write to your state and federal representatives.

A good way to get their attention is to be brief and direct. They may not spare much time reading a letter. They must decide quickly where and how their time is best spent. Here is a letter to grab their attention and fill in your concerns.

Dear Representative _____,

If we are expected to live with 21st century medicine, let us have 21st century laws. If we are to experiment with capitalistic approaches to medicine, please be reasonable with patients' rights. Innovation and progress are not the problems, but some important details are missing.

1.
2.
3.

Thank you for your attention to these matters.

Sincerely,

Governments should be supported so long as its ends are morally correct. When they are not, the wise minority must resist by urging that government revise public policy. Thoreau refused to pay taxes to support a government that ignores a majority's rights. This, he calls, is the duty of civil disobedience. The concept was used by Gandhi, Martin Luther King, and others. Must we become this desperate before attention is given to the needs of the voters?

Finally, I want to thank you for becoming more involved in health care. Our future health depends on what you do next.

References

Phelps, C. (1997). *Health Economics* (2nd Ed.). New York, NY: Addison-Wesley Educational Publishers, Inc.

Stigler, G. (1971). "The Theory of Economic Regulation." *The Bell Journal of Economics and Management Science 2,* (1), 3–21.

Index

A
accountability, 32, 142, 145, 151
actuary, 88-89
acupuncture, 129
adverse outcomes, 66, 88-89
AIDS, 35, 57, 72, 139
alcohol, 36, 110, 136, 140
alternative therapies, 111, 128, 151
appeals, 10, 75, 151
arbitration, 49
assisted living, 127-128, 147
asthma, 12, 61, 98
asymmetric information, 72-73, 104
authorization, 74
autonom, 103y
avoidance, 101, 113

B
beneficence, 92, 103
benefits, 18, 138, 139, 141, 145
bone marrow transplants, 138
bounty hunting, 58-59
breast cancer, 86
Britain, 154

C
Canada, 95, 113, 114, 115, 116, 120, 150, 154
cancer, 35, 57, 72, 98, 138
capitation, 19, 35, 40, 55, 57, 61, 88, 89, 102, 103, 106, 126
cardiac catheterization, 112
case management, 61, 63-64, 68
case manager, 63-71, 74, 145
catastrophe, 107
catch-up economics, 28
Cesarean section, 86

children, 105, 109, 138
chiropractic, 129, 146
cholesterol, 134, 136, 137
chronic illness, 33, 34, 35, 36, 57, 78, 79, 81, 98, 99
clinical trials, 10, 59-60, 151
Colorado, 42, 96
community, 53, 55, 127
competition, 7, 41, 53, 56, 95, 99, 127, 153
complaints, 10, 31
confidentiality, 10, 92, 127
conflict of interest, 101, 102-103, 117, 152
consumer awareness, 111, 126-127
consumerism, 9-11, 26, 105, 106, 108, 109, 143, 154-155
contract, 31, 32, 33, 47, 112, 118
cooperative care, 33-36
co-payment, 22, 74, 150
cost containment, 28, 29, 35, 39, 63, 132, 133
cost-effective analysis, 134, 135, 137-139, 141coverage, 11, 118, 119. *See also* universal coverage

D
demand, 25-26, 73, 78, 79, 111, 147, 153
dental, 121
diabetes, 34, 86, 98
Diagnostic Related Groupings (DRGs), 12, 13, 63, 65, 66, 69, 70, 147
diluted coverage, 60, 74, 75
disability, 82, 99
disease management, 61, 63, 70, 72

disclosure, 151
discounts, 55, 58
disincentives, 22, 32, 58, 152, 153
doctors. *See* physicians
downsizing, 12-14
drugs, 36, 50, 110, 134, 140

E

economies of scale, 53, 55, 90
efficiency, 72, 79, 80, 81, 84, 90, 111, 112, 113, 121
elderly, 7, 12, 17, 78, 79, 109, 118, 127, 138, 147, 153
emergencies, 10, 24, 31, 79, 136, 151
employees, 7, 15, 21, 32, 44, 47, 57, 58, 73, 107, 117, 118, 126
employers, 7, 15, 17, 21, 23, 25, 30, 31, 32, 40, 44-52, 55, 57, 58, 83, 84, 86, 104, 107, 113, 114, 117, 118, 126, 127, 131
equity, 72, 84, 121
ERISA, 10, 21, 23, 46, 47, 49, 101, 114
ethics, 91, 92, 97, 144
Exclusive Provider Organization, 56
externalities, 109

F

federal bill of rights, 17, 18-19
federal perspective, 72-83
fee-for-service, 11, 13, 16, 18, 25, 28, 29, 48, 56, 61, 102, 103, 104, 110, 147, 150
fidelity, 92
formularies, 10, 152
for-profit, 41, 43, 53, 59, 94, 116, 147
free riders, 60, 139

G

gag clause, 60, 72, 101, 120
gatekeeping, 24, 27, 35, 45, 74, 77, 78, 80, 102, 103, 112, 120, 140
geographically specific solutions, 101, 151
good faith, 92, 103, 105
group model HMOs, 56

H

Hawaii, 114, 115
health care, 7, 8, 13, 14, 16-21, 22, 24
Health Care Financing Administration (HCFA), 45
health care resources, 42
health insurance, 17, 19, 39, 49, 66, 82, 83, 103
health plans or policies, 7, 40, 41, 106
heart disease, 34, 65, 98, 134
HEDIS (Health Plan Employer Data and Information Set), 85, 86, 120
high risk, 57, 82, 110, 127, 134, 151, 154
history, 11-12
HIV. *See* AIDs
HMOs
    common types, 56
    defined, 9-15
    how they work, 14, 28
    physician-sponsored, 30, 36
    provider-sponsored HMOs, 31, 101, 103-105
home health care, 22, 55, 63, 121, 138, 142, 143
hospital(s), 11, 12, 13, 14, 18, 20, 23, 30, 32, 38-43, 46, 48, 49, 53, 55, 57, 58, 61, 62, 63, 64, 68, 70, 75, 81, 88, 89, 90, 91, 95, 97, 101, 104, 106, 117, 123, 125, 142, 143, 145
    physician-sponsored, 30
    provider-sponsored, 31
hospital network, physician-sponsored, 38-40
hospital's perspective, 38-43
human resources, 42

I

immunization, 86, 105, 121, 126
incentives, 19, 22, 25, 26, 28, 32, 39, 55, 56, 61, 80, 81, 95, 96, 97, 103, 105, 107, 112, 113, 150, 152
Independent Practice Association, 56
indigent, 18, 38, 41
informed consent, 60

inpatient services, 24, 46, 58, 63, 80, 138, 143
integrated delivery systems, 53, 127, 142

J
justice, 92, 96, 103, 145

K
Kennedy-Kassenbaum, 82
kidney dialysis,. 97
kidney transplant, 97, 138

L
lawsuits, 11, 34, 49
legislators, 12, 16, 42, 46, 48, 49, 152, 154
litigation, 34, 75, 92

M
malpractice, 33, 44, 49, 91
mammography, 143
managed care, 7, 14, 16-21, 24, 28, 29, 32, 36, 38, 39, 40, 41, 42, 45, 53-62, 63, 75, 84, 86, 87, 88, 89, 90, 93, 95, 102, 103, 105, 116, 125, 126, 129, 131, 132, 139
managed competition, 55-56
mastectomy, 10
mayo clinic, 30, 31, 104
Medicaid, 7, 11, 12, 17, 20, 21, 35, 42, 44, 45, 50, 51, 63, 75, 82, 97, 127
medical Savings Accounts (MSAs), 25, 26, 95, 101, 106-113, 115, 136, 145, 147, 154
Medicare, 7, 11, 12, 13, 17, 19, 21, 35, 42, 44, 45, 51, 63, 75, 76, 77, 78, 79, 80, 81, 82, 118, 127, 147, 153
mental health, 112
mergers & acquisitions, 125
Minnesota, 30, 115
mixed model HMOs, 56
monitors, 61-62, 103, 136, 137
monopoly, 20, 36, 40, 55, 80, 104, 110
moral hazard, 48, 78, 79, 81, 97, 111, 134, 145

N
National Committee for Quality Assurance (NCQA), 66, 67, 68, 85, 86, 120
network(s), 14, 24, 42, 55, 66, 68, 79, 88, 89, 91, 103
    provider-sponsored, 103, 104, 112, 115
non-maleficence, 92, 103, 129, 145
not-for-profit, 41, 53, 115
nurse practitioners, 29, 34, 64, 68, 75, 76, 77, 78, 79, 80, 81, 111, 147, 153

O
opportunity costs, 109, 134, 136, 138, 140
ophthalmology, 144
organ donation, 95-99
outcomes, 85-89, 95, 105

P
patients, 11, 12, 13, 14, 18, 20, 21, 22, 23, 25, 27, 28, 29, 31, 32, 33, 34, 35, 36, 40, 41, 42, 46, 48, 49, 52, 55, 56, 59, 60, 61, 64, 66, 70, 72, 73, 76, 77, 78, 79, 81, 84, 85, 86, 87, 88, 89, 90, 91, 94, 95, 97, 101, 102, 103, 105, 108, 110, 111, 112, 113, 116, 123, 127, 128, 129, 131, 135, 144, 145, 151, 153, 154
patient satisfaction, 61, 86, 87
physical herapy, 64, 65, 144
physician(s), 7, 11, 12, 13, 18, 23, 25, 27-36, 40, 53, 55, 56, 57, 58, 59, 60, 61, 62, 69, 70, 74, 75, 76, 77, 78, 79, 80, 81, 82, 97, 102, 103, 104, 105, 110, 115, 117, 118, 126, 136, 137, 140, 145, 146, 147
Physician-Hospital Organization, 56
point-of-service plan, 56
poverty patients, 7, 44, 45, 46, 47, 65, 147, 153
Preferred Provider Organizations, 56
pregnancy, 36, 127, 134, 137
premium, 20, 98, 100, 104, 107, 114,

116, 127, 150, 154
prescription, 108, 121
prevention, 80, 81, 85, 91, 95, 108, 109, 116, 117, 118, 126
primary care, 75, 78, 80, 81, 85, 116
primary care physician, 27, 28, 45
protocols, 61, 62, 65-66, 67, 68, 70, 74, 75, 90, 93, 126, 127, 140, 145, 152
provider(s), 7, 11, 14, 18, 20, 39, 46, 57, 58, 61, 66, 72, 74, 79, 85, 89, 90, 91, 92, 93, 101, 102, 103, 104, 106, 108, 110, 111, 117, 118, 121, 123, 125, 126, 128, 129, 137, 140, 142, 146, 151
providers' perspective, 27-36
purchasing cooperatives, 20

Q

quality, 42, 43, 49, 53, 61, 66, 67, 74, 77, 87, 90, 101, 111, 112, 114, 117, 144-145

R

rationing, 24, 25, 27, 31, 41, 42, 50, 60, 73-76, 78, 81, 95, 101, 106, 109, 111, 120, 137, 140, 144, 154
rational behavior, 22-23
referral, 74
regulatory agencies, 152
rehabilitation, 144
reimbursement, 73, 76, 80
report cards, 86, 87
research, 61
respect, 61
right, 16, 17
responsibility, 16, 17, 67, 151

S

screening, 84
second opinion, 109, 142
self-ration, 31, 95, 137, 145
Smith, Adam, 94-95, 96, 106, 112
smoking, 66, 86, 136, 140
social costs, 77, 109, 134, 140
specialist, 10, 27, 57, 77, 78, 96, 112, 114
staff model HMO, 56

state bill of rights, 19-21, 46
state innovations, 45-46
states' perspective, 14, 44-52
statins, 134-136, 137, 140
supply, 24, 73, 78, 79, 147, 153

T

technology, 39
treatment, 10, 34, 61, 92, 102, 126, 135, 136, 139

U

universal access, 18
universal coverage, 16, 101, 110, 116-120, 147
utilization, 88, 152

V

vaccines, 34
veracity, 92, 103
Viagra, 134, 136
vitamins, 129

W

Wisconsin, 50, 51, 53, 54
women, 50, 51

Y

yin and yang, 38, 43

Related Books by The Crossing Press

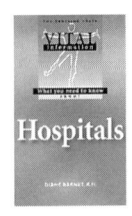

Hospitals
By Diane Barnet, R.N.

Hospitals can be intimidating places. Many consumers don't know how to obtain information or even what questions to ask. *Hospitals* provides inside information for patients and their advocates, and will help you deal with hospitals as a well-informed consumer.

$11.95 • Paper • ISBN 0-89594-908-3

Perimenopause
By Bernard Cortese, M.D.

Perimenopause is the word that refers to the transitional time before and after menopause. This book describes the changes that may take place, discusses the pros and cons of hormone replacement therapy (HRT), offers alternative treatments, and stresses the importance of exercise, proper diet, and stress management.

$11.95 • Paper • ISBN 0-89594-914-8

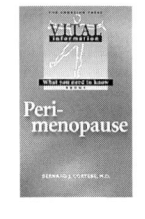

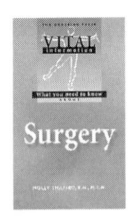

Surgery
By Molly Shapiro, R.N., M.S.-M.B.A., Ed.D

Surgery covers every aspect of the surgery process including what your rights are as a patient. It tells you how to prepare for surgery, what happens in surgery, explains equipment use and procedures, and answers your post-op concerns.

$11.95 • Paper • ISBN 0-89594-898-2

Vitamins, Minerals & Supplements
By Gayle Skowronski and Beth Petro Roybal

Vitamins, Minerals & Supplements gives general information about the role of supplements in nutrition and how to choose them wisely. It gives details for specific common nutritional supplements and the daily requirements necessary to maintain good health.

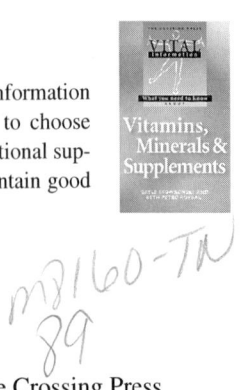

$11.95 • Paper • ISBN 0-89594-935-0

To receive a current catalog from The Crossing Press
please call toll-free, 800-777-1048.
Visit our Web site: **www.crossingpress.com**